Well done.

You have just undergone the most physically and emotionally exhausting process of your life.

You have successfully subdivided.

You have a baby.

You can take it home with you.

Unlike a library book, which you have to return after three weeks, this child is yours for years and years.

But what do you do with it?

What next?

In our society, you are unlikely to have lived with any other breastfeeding mothers.

You don't see breastfeeding on the telly.

Many people are too shy to breastfeed in public.

Chances are, your mother didn't breastfeed.

Over a third of new mothers who try breastfeeding don't really get the hang of it, and give up in the first six weeks.[1]

HELP!

Help!

We used to be really good at breastfeeding! Women have been suckling their young for two million years. Look how successful we've been at propagating the human race (6 billion and counting…). If we hadn't been breastfeeding for all that time, there wouldn't have been anyone around to invent formula milk.

Breastfeeding feels very nice! It's a beautiful, intimately connected way to communicate with your baby.

Now this book doesn't have all the answers. This is *your* baby, who isn't the same as the one in the books. You will arrive naturally at your own style of parenting, and feel free to take any advice about babycare, including all of this, with a pinch of salt.

Still, you will find all the information here you might need to help you breastfeed successfully.

And, if you're feeling too brain-dead for reading, there are loads of pictures to look at instead. Great!

The Food of Love

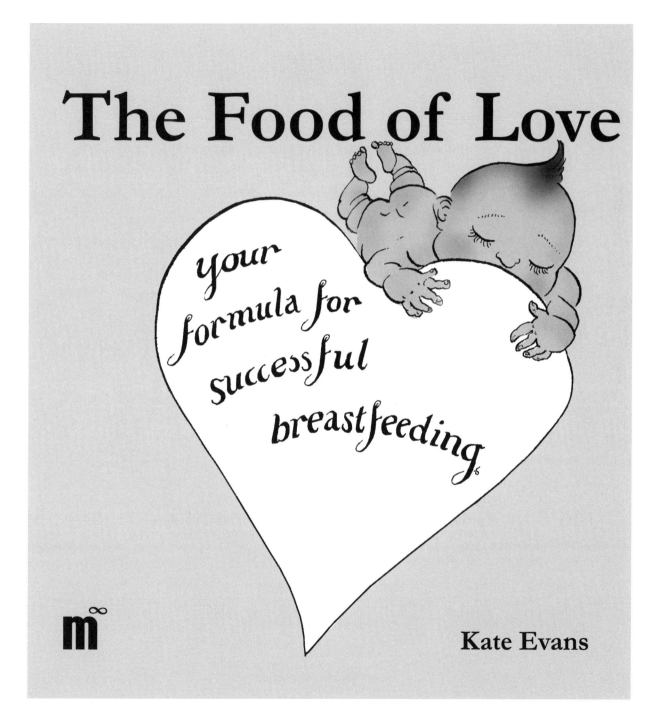

your formula for successful breastfeeding

m∞

Kate Evans

First published in 2009 by

Myriad Editions
New Internationalist
The Old Music Hall
106–108 Cowley Road
Oxford OX4 1JE

www.MyriadEditions.com

Reprinted 2010, 2011, 2012, 2013, 2014, 2015, 2017, 2018

Ninth printing

Copyright © Kate Evans 2009, 2015

The moral right of the author has been asserted.

Every effort has been made to obtain the necessary permissions
with reference to copyright material; should there be any omissions
we apologize and shall be pleased to make the appropriate
acknowledgements in any future edition.

The New Contented Little Baby Book by Gina Ford (Vermilion).
Reprinted by permission of The Random House Group Ltd.

What to Expect When You're Breastfeeding…and What if You Can't?
by Clare Byam-Cook (Vermilion). Reprinted by permission of
The Random House Group Ltd.

The Physical Life of Man and Woman by Pye Henry Chavasse MD
(National Publishing Company, Ohio, 1872)

Chambers' Encyclopaedia vol 10 (Chambers, 1880)

Mr Chambers' Cyclopædia by Ephraim Chambers
ed. George Lewis Scott (Chambers, 1753)

All rights reserved. No part of this publication may be reproduced,
stored in a retrieval system, or transmitted in any form or by any
means without the written permission of the publisher, nor be
otherwise circulated in any form of binding or cover other than that
in which it is published and without a similar condition including
this condition being imposed on the subsequent purchaser.

A CIP catalogue record for this book is available from
the British Library.

ISBN (pbk): 978-0-9549309-5-0
ISBN (ebk): 978-1-908434-83-8

Designed by Kate Evans

Follow *The Food of Love* on Facebook

Printed in Poland on paper sourced from sustainable forests.
www.lfbookservices.co.uk

Contents

Foreword:
A community midwife writes...

As a community midwife a large and rewarding part of my job involves helping and advising new parents throughout the early days of breastfeeding. When I leave them, I often feel worried that I am abandoning them to another sleepless and anxious night with little support and a punishing regime to fulfil. Of course my aim is to make things easier and facilitate blissful breastfeeding for many months. However, that first couple of weeks can be tricky.

I often wish I could leave a breastfeeding support worker to help them through those initial few days of latching problems or jaundice or non-stop suckling.

Hooray! Kate's book is the closest companion to a 24-hour breastfeeding support worker that I can imagine. What's more, it will make you laugh, which is essential when new parenthood is overwhelming you. I only wish the NHS could afford to hand out copies so that when I turn up at people's houses to find shell-shocked, brand-new parents with huge black-ringed eyes and hair that looks like it's just been through a wind tunnel saying 'believe me, this is the first time that baby has slept since you left yesterday!' I could give them a copy of *The Food of Love* to advise, reassure and entertain them.

Breastfeeding does just happen for the lucky few, but the majority of new mums, even those who have successfully breastfed before, will need a little support to get started. It is important not to feel isolated and anxious. I believe a huge source of anxiety is the belief that everyone else is blissfully breastfeeding like professionals and you are the only mummy and baby that seem to be struggling. I can say that all the situations which Kate describes are common and occur frequently amongst my clients.

In a world which is becoming increasingly better-informed about health, nutrition and well-being, from birth to school dinners, breastfeeding is indisputably the best possible start in life that you can give your baby. This book can help more mums to establish and enjoy the bliss of happily breastfeeding their babies for as long as they wish to. It is an essential read for the 21st-century mum.

—Ali Dale, RM

What are breasts?

mine are too big

mine are too small

my nipples are too pointy
and they show through
my clothes

my nipples are too flat
they look weird

mine are too droopy

mine are odd sizes

I don't know about you, but the first thing I felt about my breasts was anxiety, because they weren't there yet, followed rapidly by embarrassment, because they were. Acquiring breasts is the obvious sign of becoming a woman – far *too* obvious for many eleven-year-old girls. Breasts in our culture are seen not as maternal but as sexual.

Breasts are sexy. Open any newspaper, look on any advertising hoarding and you'll see breasts performing their primary function: looking nice for men to get excited about.

It follows, therefore, that as sex organs, breasts should be kept private, and certainly not put in babies' mouths. That's kind of...unnatural!

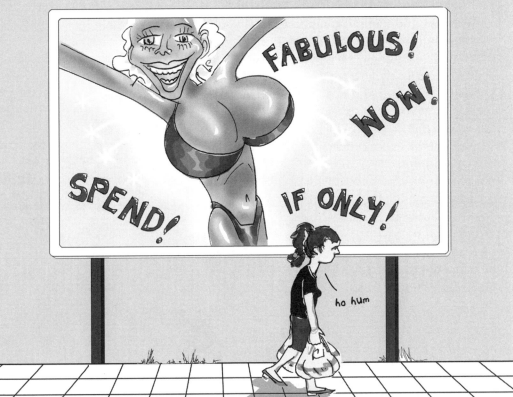

FABULOUS!

NOW!

SPEND!

IF ONLY!

ho hum

Most of the rest of the world think we're mad.

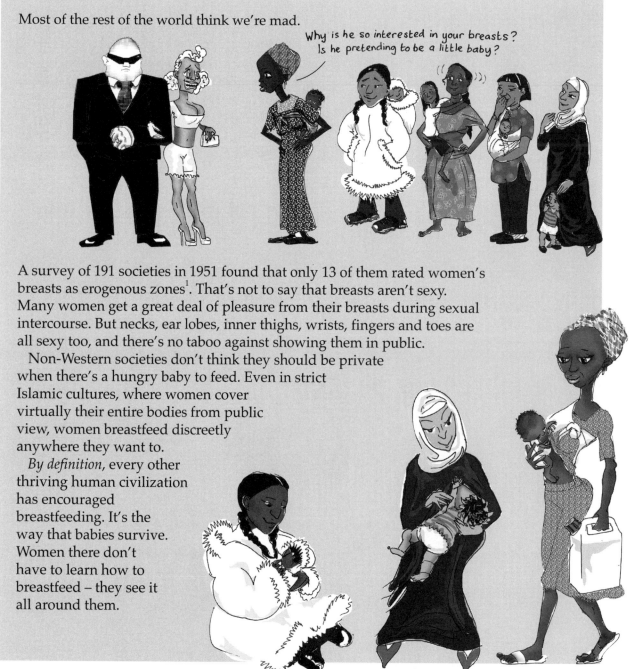

Why is he so interested in your breasts? Is he pretending to be a little baby?

A survey of 191 societies in 1951 found that only 13 of them rated women's breasts as erogenous zones[1]. That's not to say that breasts aren't sexy. Many women get a great deal of pleasure from their breasts during sexual intercourse. But necks, ear lobes, inner thighs, wrists, fingers and toes are all sexy too, and there's no taboo against showing them in public.

Non-Western societies don't think they should be private when there's a hungry baby to feed. Even in strict Islamic cultures, where women cover virtually their entire bodies from public view, women breastfeed discreetly anywhere they want to.

By definition, every other thriving human civilization has encouraged breastfeeding. It's the way that babies survive. Women there don't have to learn how to breastfeed – they see it all around them.

Still, here we are in the West. Our tribal support networks have vanished. We are split up into flats and houses, embarking alone on the experience of mothering, something that society views as a temporary career break. And breasts, here, are sexy. Breastfeeding seems weird. Bottlefeeding seems easier. Babies miss out.

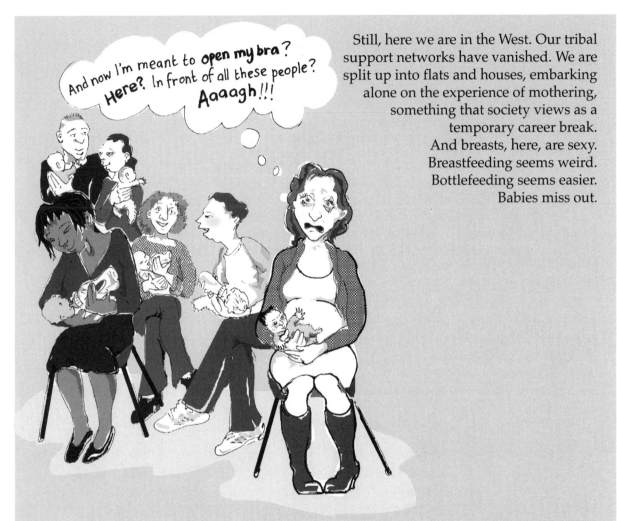

You are much less likely to breastfeed if all your friends' babies are bottle-fed.

This is a shame. Breastfeeding is lovely. Babies love it. Mothers love it. Your body is capable of producing this amazing, perfect food that will transform your tiny baby into the happiest, cleverest, healthiest kid they can be.

And it's free! Breastmilk is so special; it would cost hundreds of pounds if you could buy it in a tin.

It's got to be worth a go.

Breasts make milk. That's what they do.

Internally, the breast looks like a tree, or a bush. You will have an average of nine milk glands or lobes in each breast – some women have more, some have fewer. Each has a duct that leads back from the nipple and divides off into what looks like branches and twigs. The 'leaves' are the alveoli, little round pockets which are lined with lactocytes, the milk-producing cells.

Around the outside of your milk gland 'tree' there are 'clouds' of fat, and there are some streaks of fat between the branches too. This means that you can't tell how big your milk glands are by looking at your breast. The size of your breast does not determine how much milk you make. That depends on how often and how much your baby drinks.

The hormone prolactin in your bloodstream triggers the lactocytes to start producing milk. As they fill up, the alveoli stretch and change the shape of the lactocytes so they can't absorb any more prolactin. So as your breasts become 'full', milk production slows down.

There is also a protein in breastmilk with the snappy name of 'Feedback Inhibitor of Breastmilk'. When the alveoli fill with milk, more and more of this protein collects there, and this also gives the lactocytes the message to stop producing milk.

Once the baby starts suckling, a rush of the hormone oxytocin makes muscles around the alveoli contract, forcing the milk down into the ducts. They swell behind the nipple, until they look like the trunk of a tree. The wave-like motion of the baby's tongue against those fat milk ducts brings big gulps of breastmilk into his mouth. The baby must get a good mouthful of breast to be able to reach the milk ducts and feed efficiently.

As the alveoli empty out, prolactin floods back into the lactocytes, so milk production starts up again. Now the baby starts to feed more slowly, and the milk that is produced becomes higher in fat and more satisfying. Once the baby has had enough of this high-fat milk, he ends the feed.

Your breasts are not like a bottle. They do not fill up with milk, then empty as a baby feeds. Your breasts are like a factory. The more your baby feeds, the more milk they make. When you let your baby feed frequently, your breasts become better at making milk. When you let him feed until he's full, you help him get the most from every feed.

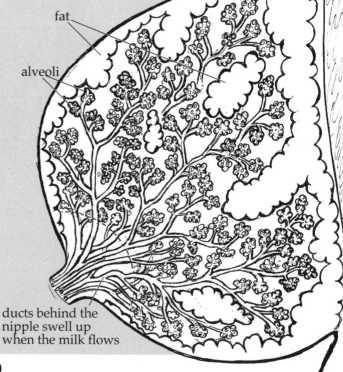

fat

alveoli

ducts behind the nipple swell up when the milk flows

What's so special about breastmilk anyway?

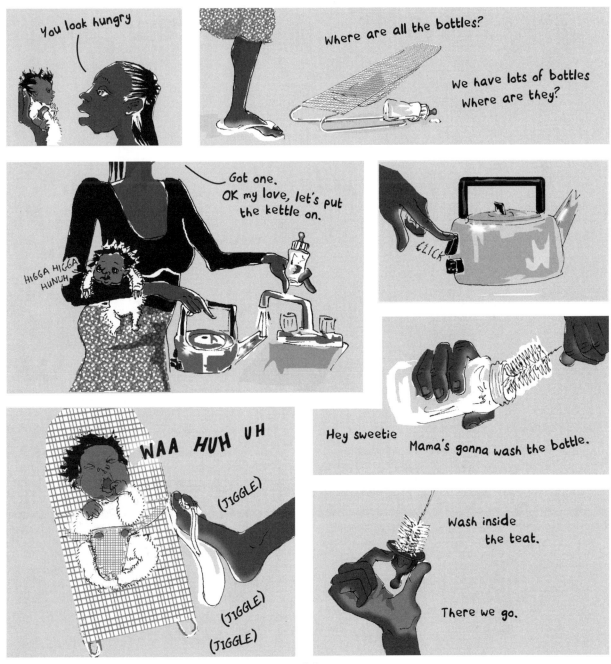

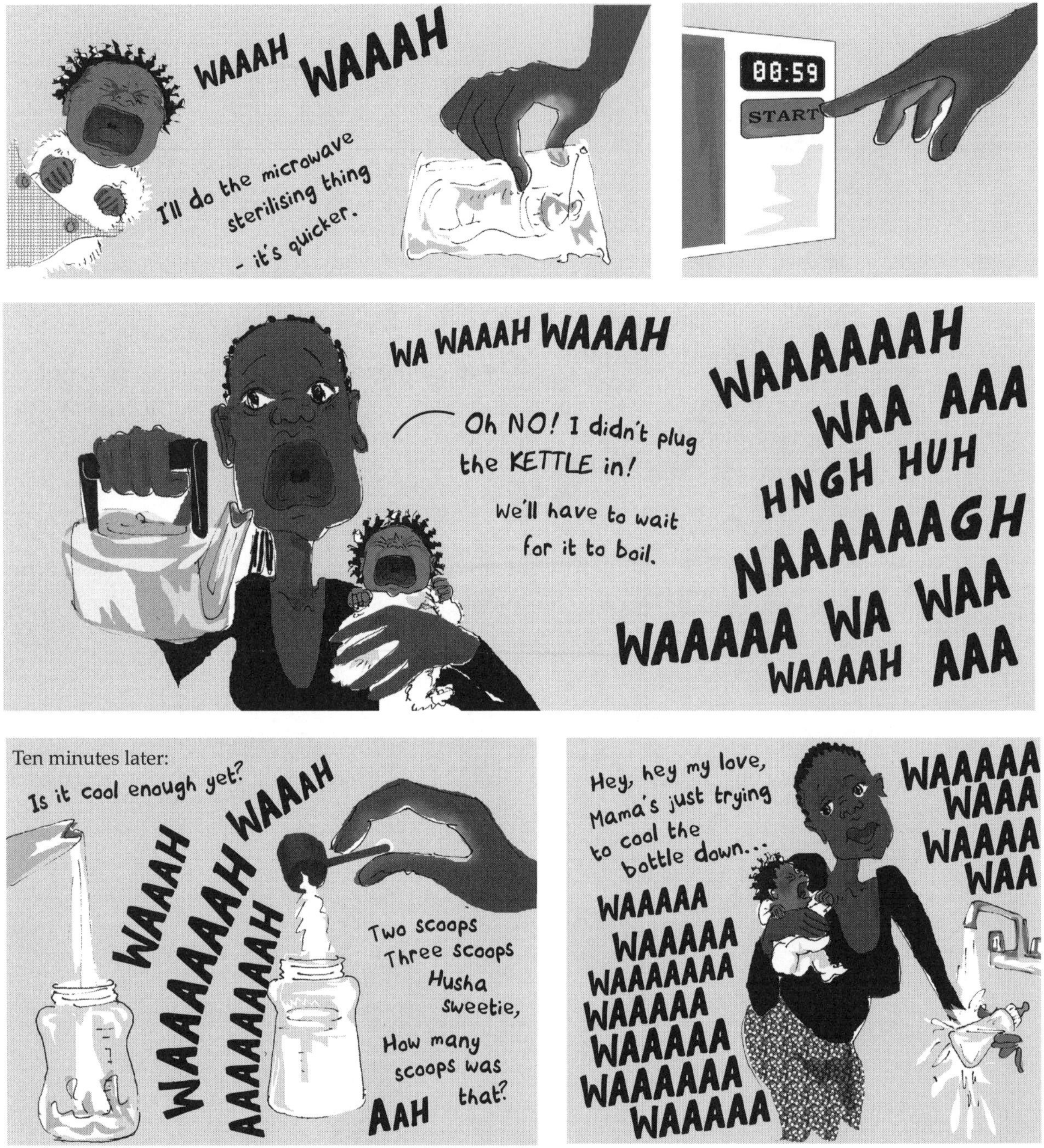
WAAAH WAAAH
I'll do the microwave sterilising thing - it's quicker.
00:59
START
WA WAAAH WAAAH
Oh NO! I didn't plug the KETTLE in!
We'll have to wait for it to boil.
WAAAAAAH
WAA AAA
HNGH HUH
NAAAAAAGH
WAAAAA WA WAA
WAAAAH AAA
Ten minutes later:
Is it cool enough yet?
WAAAH
WAAAAAAH WAAAH
AAAAAAAAH
Two scoops
Three scoops
Husha sweetie,
How many scoops was that?
AAH
Hey, hey my love, Mama's just trying to cool the bottle down...
WAAAAA
WAAA
WAAAA
WAA
WAAAAA
WAAAAA
WAAAAAAA
WAAAAA
WAAAAA
WAAAAAA
WAAAAA

You look hungry.
Breastfeeding is easy!

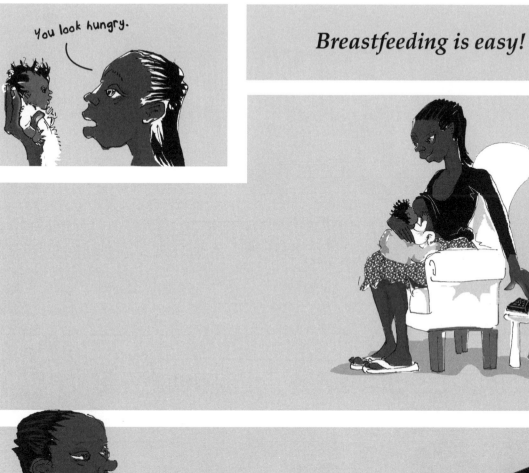

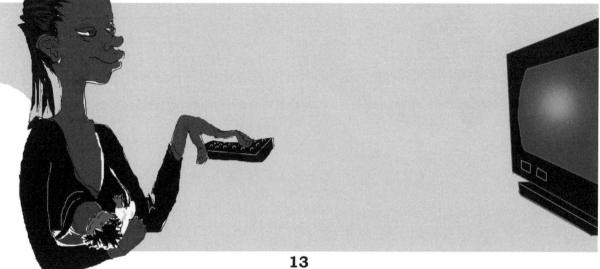

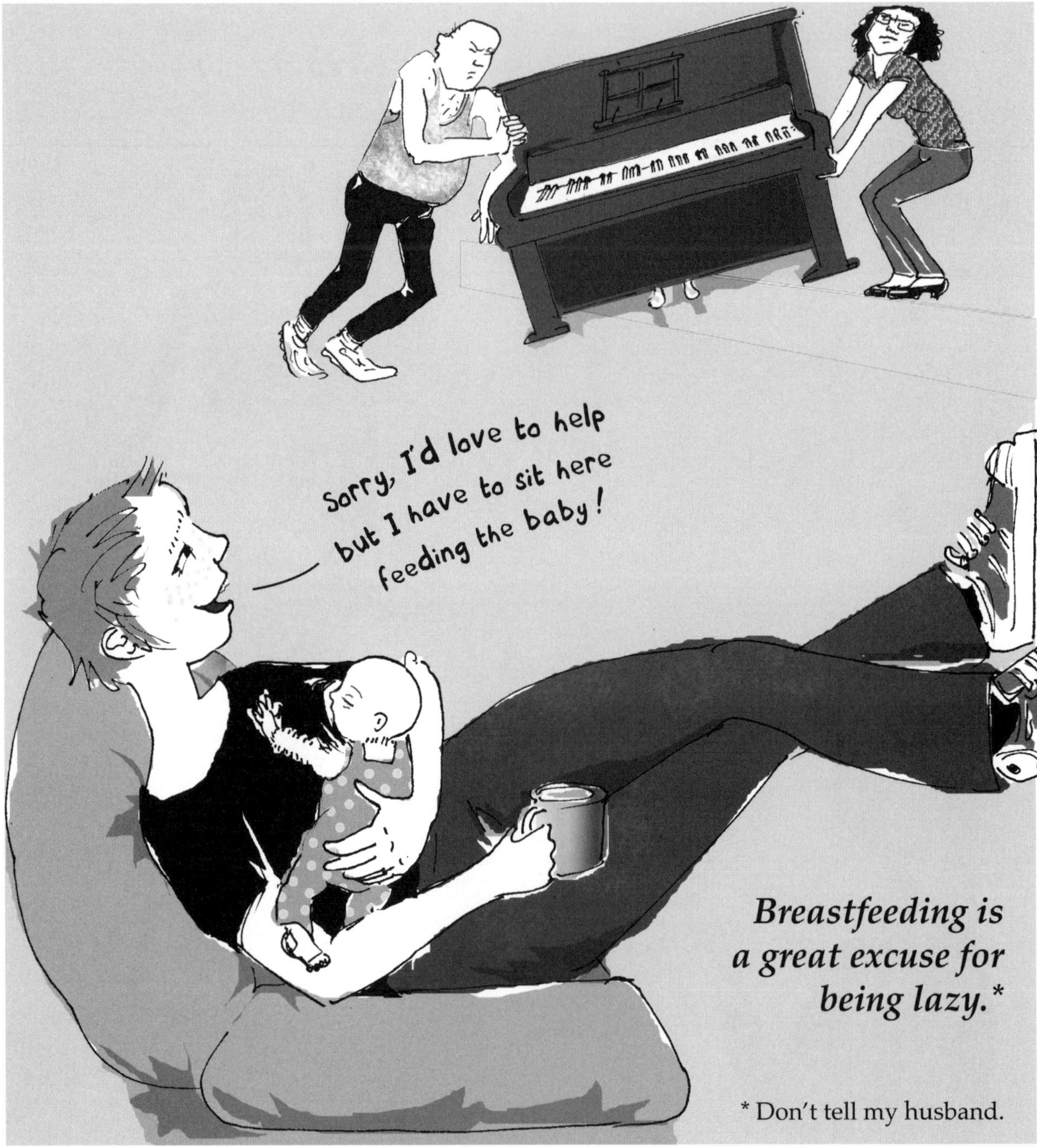
Sorry, I'd love to help
but I have to sit here
feeding the baby!

*Breastfeeding is a great excuse for being lazy.**

* Don't tell my husband.

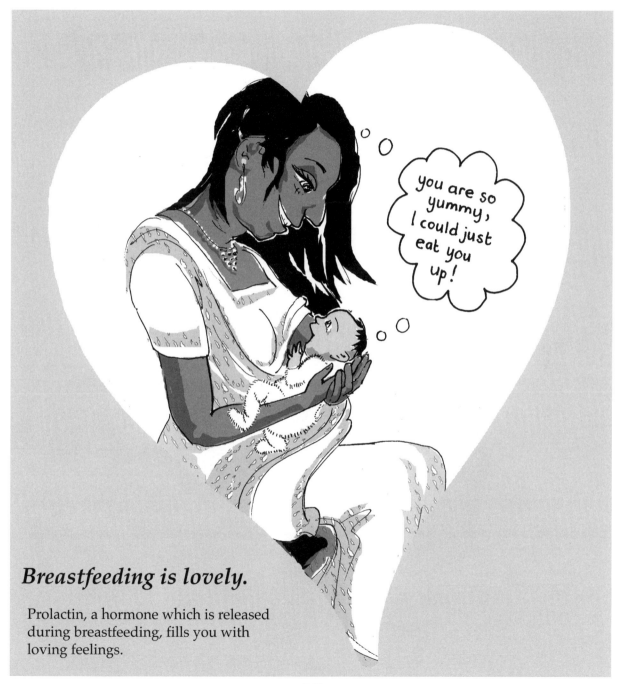

Breastfeeding is lovely.

Prolactin, a hormone which is released during breastfeeding, fills you with loving feelings.

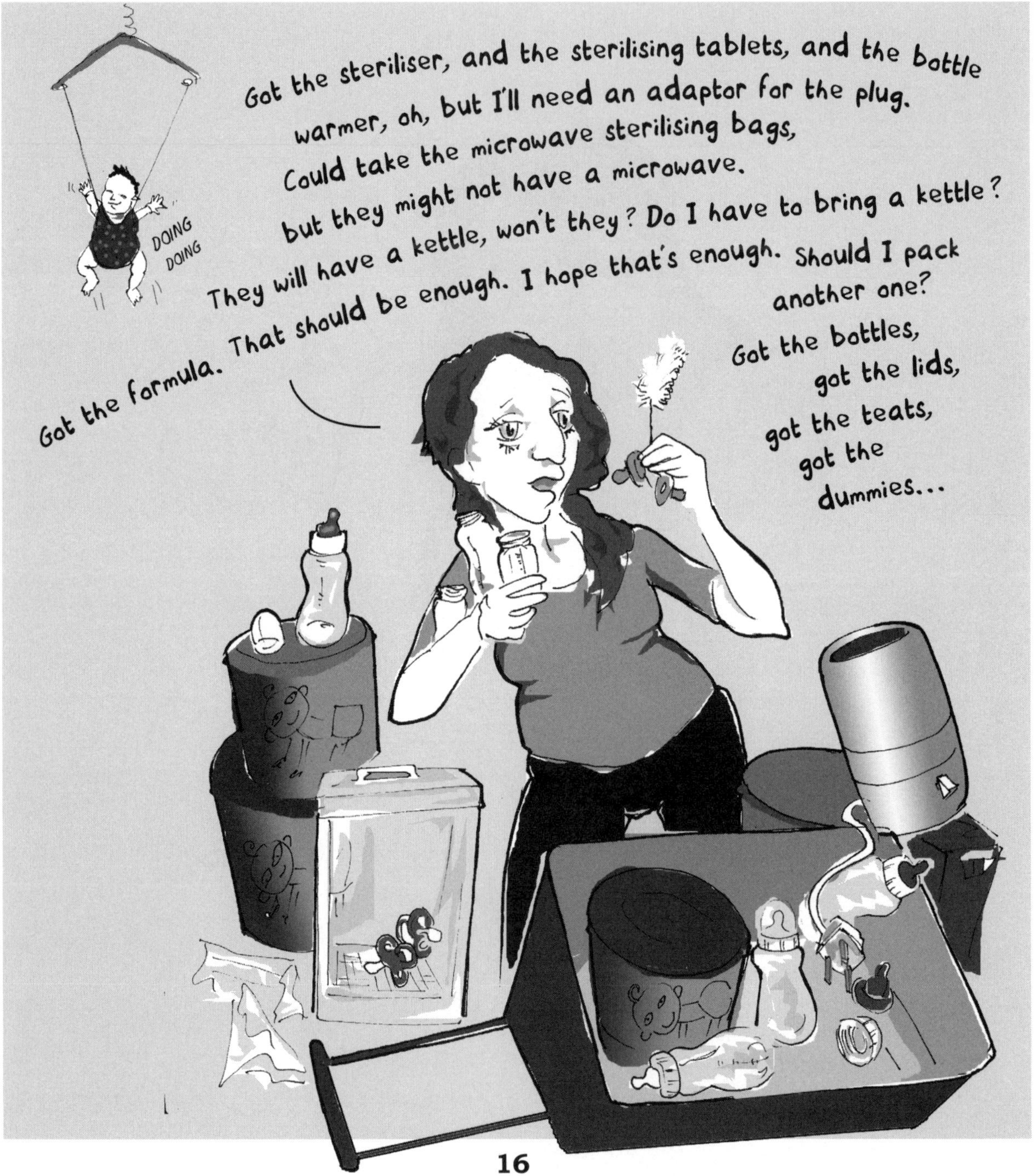
DOING
DOING
Got the steriliser, and the sterilising tablets, and the bottle
warmer, oh, but I'll need an adaptor for the plug.
Could take the microwave sterilising bags,
but they might not have a microwave.
They will have a kettle, won't they? Do I have to bring a kettle?
Got the formula. That should be enough. I hope that's enough. Should I pack another one?
Got the bottles,
got the lids,
got the teats,
got the dummies...

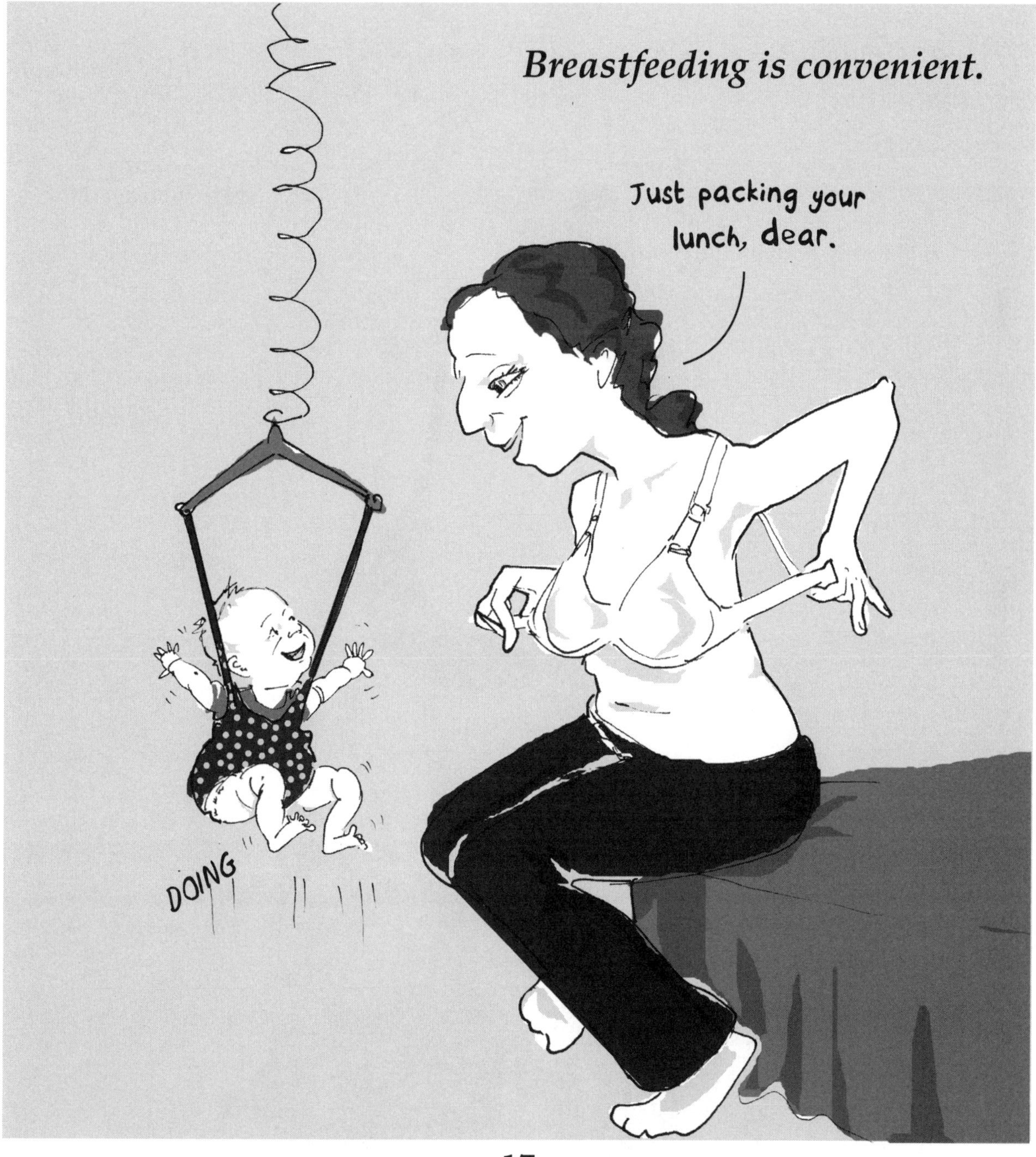
Just packing your lunch, dear.
DOING

Breastfeeding is convenient.

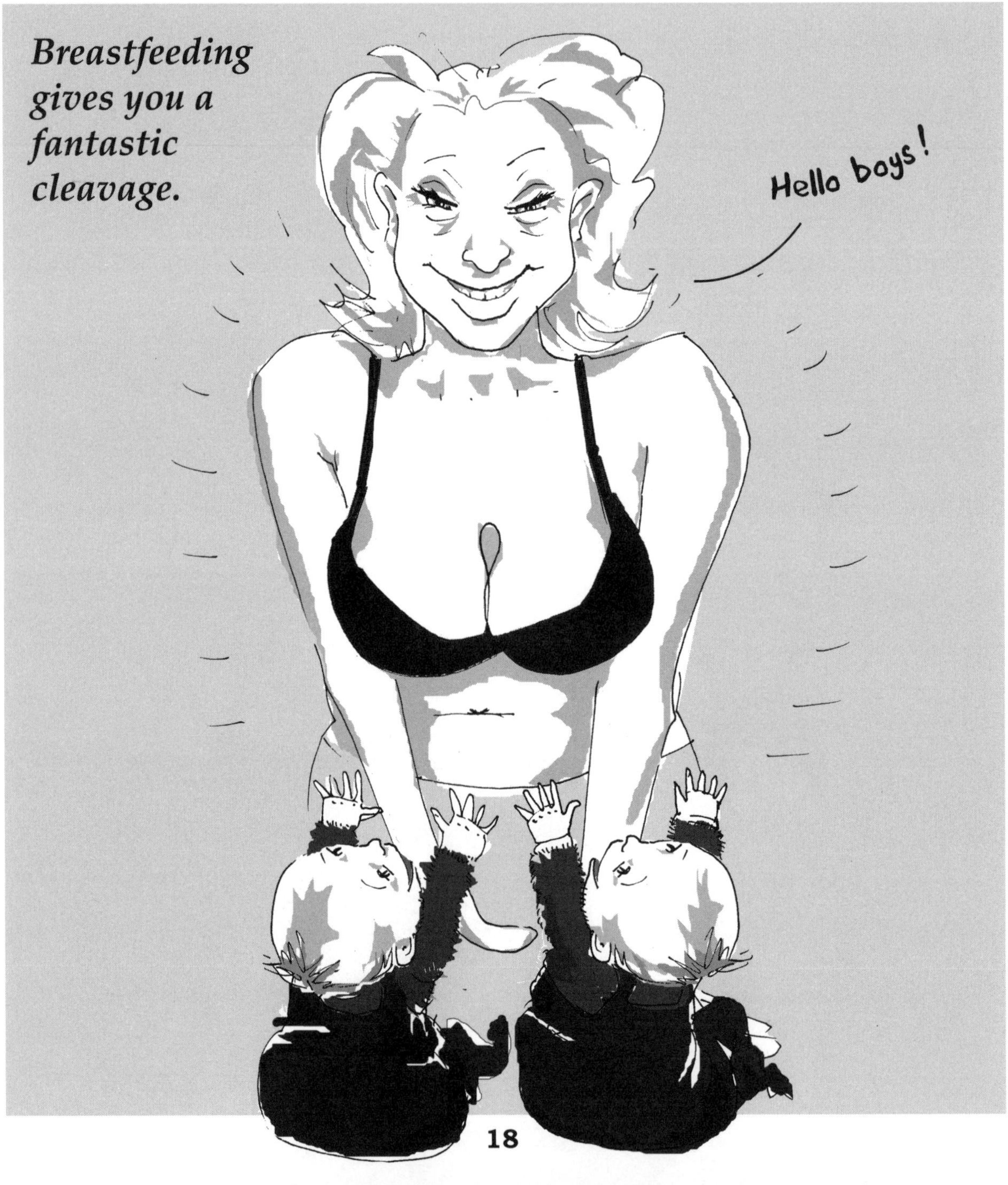
Breastfeeding gives you a fantastic cleavage.
Hello boys!

Breastfeeding helps you lose weight...

Or, depending on how you look at things,
breastfeeding is a brilliant excuse to
carry on eating double dinners!

*Brilliant! A thousand
extra calories every day.*

...it helps you to get back in shape...

The hormone oxytocin, which is released when a baby suckles,
also helps your womb shrink back down to size.

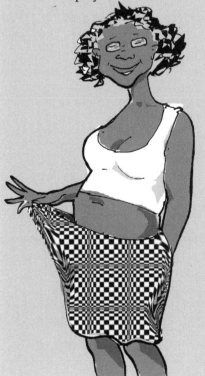

...and it protects your child against obesity.

Breastfed babies know how much to eat. The
rich, creamy hind-milk that comes at the end
of a feed contains a substance which makes
them feel naturally full. Breastfed babies are
35% less likely to become overweight
six-year-olds than babies fed on formula.[1]

Breastfed babies are cleverer.

Hmm, if I'm not mistaken this milk contains docosahexaenoic arachidonic acid, omega-3 fatty acids and optimum glucose and cholesterol levels for brain and nerve development.

It seems that scientists have still not discovered all the ways in which breastmilk aids brain growth.

Just wait 'til I grow up.

Human beings have very large brains, and human milk is the best substance for growing them. So, breastfed babies have higher IQs than formula-fed babies. And, the longer babies are breastfed, the smarter they get[2].

20

Breastfeeding helps your baby sleep.

Breastmilk contains the natural sleep promoter 'delta-sleep-inducing-peptide'[3]. Formula milk doesn't.

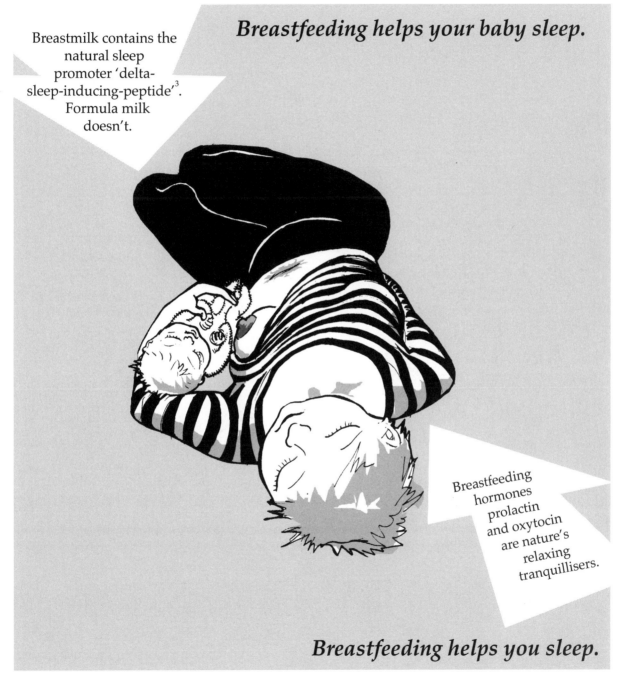

Breastfeeding hormones prolactin and oxytocin are nature's relaxing tranquillisers.

Breastfeeding helps you sleep.

21

Breastfed babies are healthier[4].

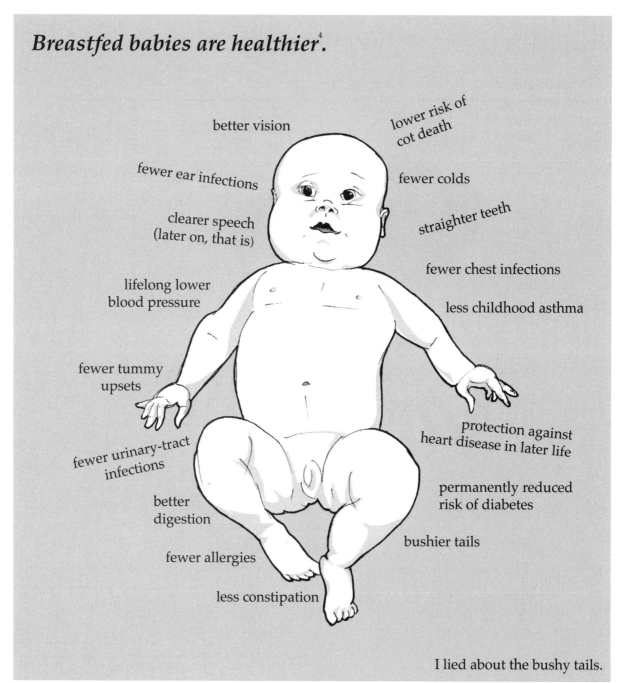

better vision

lower risk of cot death

fewer ear infections

fewer colds

clearer speech (later on, that is)

straighter teeth

fewer chest infections

lifelong lower blood pressure

less childhood asthma

fewer tummy upsets

protection against heart disease in later life

fewer urinary-tract infections

permanently reduced risk of diabetes

better digestion

bushier tails

fewer allergies

less constipation

I lied about the bushy tails.

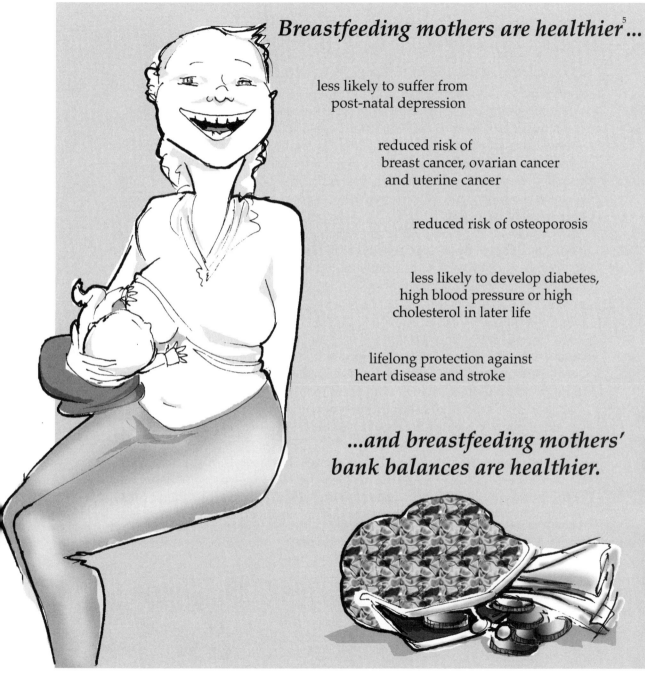

Breastfeeding mothers are healthier [5] ...

less likely to suffer from
post-natal depression

reduced risk of
breast cancer, ovarian cancer
and uterine cancer

reduced risk of osteoporosis

less likely to develop diabetes,
high blood pressure or high
cholesterol in later life

lifelong protection against
heart disease and stroke

*...and breastfeeding mothers'
bank balances are healthier.*

How does breastmilk keep your baby healthy?

Your baby does not have an efficient immune system at birth. It takes up to a year for him to start producing enough antibodies to protect himself from serious illnesses. Until then, he needs...breastmilk!

Every drop of your milk contains literally millions of white blood cells – those same white blood cells which circulate through your bloodstream, gobbling up harmful viruses and bacteria. These cells pass straight into your baby's blood and help protect him from every illness that you have ever suffered in the past.

Breastmilk also contains infection-fighting proteins known as immuno-globulins. These are like natural antibiotics which act against harmful germs that your baby may encounter, but at the same time, allow beneficial bacteria in the digestive system to flourish. Groovy, huh? Breastmilk even protects against parasites!

But this is the best bit:

The infection-fighting properties of your milk are being continually updated in response to your environment. When you encounter a new germ, your mature immune system will knock up some white blood cells to fight it off and immediately pass them to your baby through your milk. And that means that if you should come down with gastric flu, for example, provided that you are careful about hygiene, it is quite likely that your baby *won't get ill*.

And whenever your baby picks up an infection, the thin skin on your nipples allows germs in his saliva to pass directly into your bloodstream. Your immune system kicks in, manufactures a few billion white blood cells in response, and administers them back at the next feed.

Just three days of breastfeeding makes a real difference to your baby's health...

Colostrum is a thick, creamy, yellow or clear milk that you only produce for a few days after your baby is born. There may not be very much of it, but it is absolutely chock-full of antibodies and immunoglobins. It works like a natural vaccination, giving your baby instant protection against a range of diseases.

Colostrum primes a baby's digestive system to work effectively. A newborn baby's intestines are immature and porous. Particles of cow's milk or other artificial foods can pass straight through the gut lining and into the bloodstream. Colostrum is rich in growth factors which help 'seal' the lining of the gut, and speed up the growth of tiny hair-like cells that digest the food. One particular immunoglobin, Secretory IgA, forms a protective coating over the gut wall to ward off gastric infections.

As well as this, colostrum is a natural laxative. This gets waste out of your baby's system quickly, which is easier on his little liver. Breastfed babies are less likely to be jaundiced.

Your colostrum is unique. You can't buy it off the shelf, and feed it in a bottle.

...but why stop after three days?

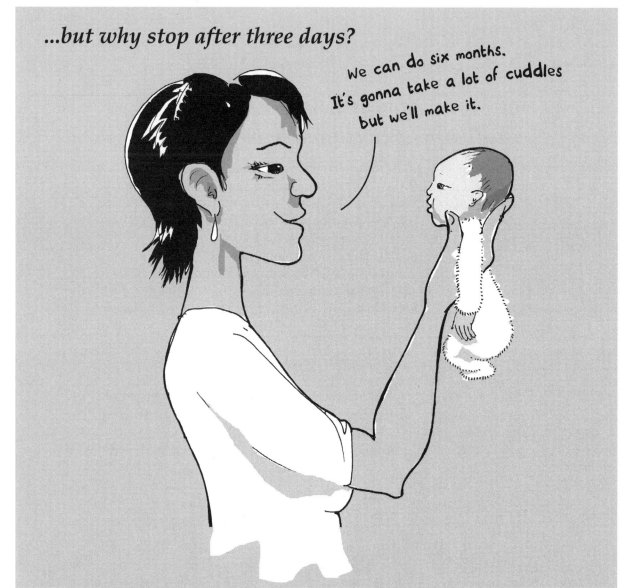

Your baby's gut matures fully at an average of about six months of age. Until the gut has matured, food particles can still 'leak' out of the gut into the bloodstream, which can trigger allergies. A baby can show you when he is ready for food by picking it up and eating it. Until then, all he needs is breastmilk.

Breastfed babies have nicer nappies.

You can smell that breastmilk is good for a baby's digestion. Breastmilk poo looks like mustard and smells like digestive biscuits.

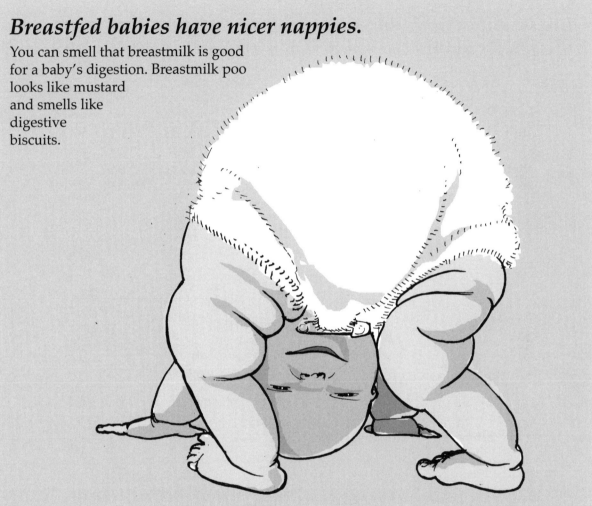

And because their urine is less acidic, they are less likely to get nappy rash.

You don't have to boil your nipples.

Nipples don't need sterilising. Don't even wash your nipples with soap, just use plain water – they keep themselves healthy and clean. By contrast, many formula-fed babies contract infections from poorly sterilised bottles or contaminated water.

Breastmilk comes in millions of varieties...

Breastmilk changes all the time. A breastfed baby gets:

A DRINK!
Thin, watery fore-milk at the beginning of each feed quenches his thirst.

A MEAL!
When he's hungry, he can carry on munching to reach the creamy, satisfying hind-milk.

SOME MEDICINE!
The latest antibodies giving protection against new germs on the scene.

NEW TASTY FLAVOURS!
Strong flavours in your food can pass into your milk and make it taste different. Babies like this, and drink more.

MORE LIQUID
WHEN IT'S NEEDED!
Your body supplies more watery fore-milk in hot weather, so you don't have to give a breastfed baby bottles of boiled water.

MORE CALORIES
WHEN THEY'RE NEEDED!
The mothers of premature babies produce more high-energy colostrum, and for longer, to help their babies thrive.

Breastmilk changes automatically; you don't have to do anything. Just sit back and enjoy it. Because there's one variety which breastmilk always comes in...

...breastmilk always comes in cuddles.

Breastmilk tastes like warm vanilla ice-cream.

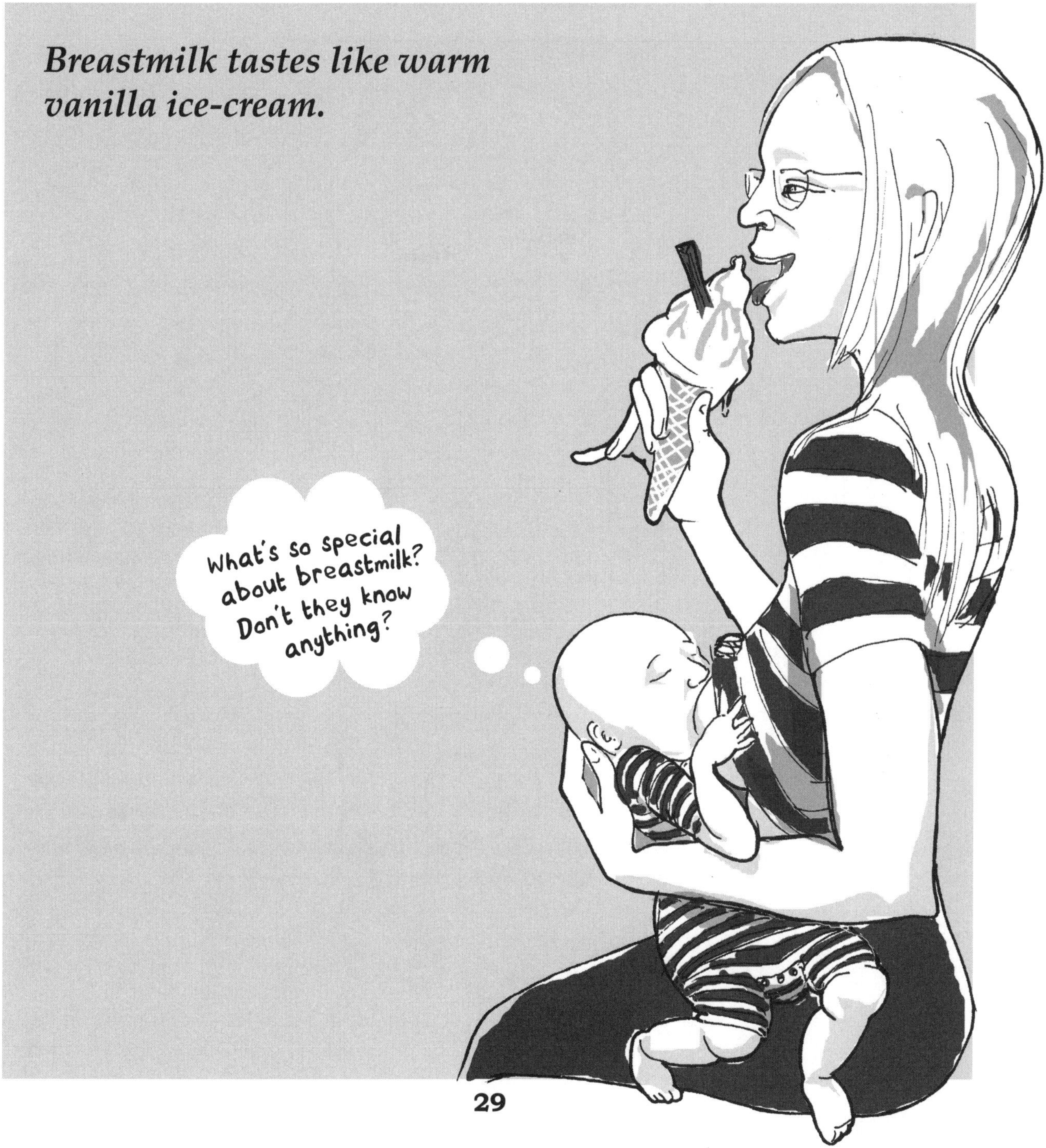
What's so special about breastmilk? Don't they know anything?

Anatomy of a Newborn Baby

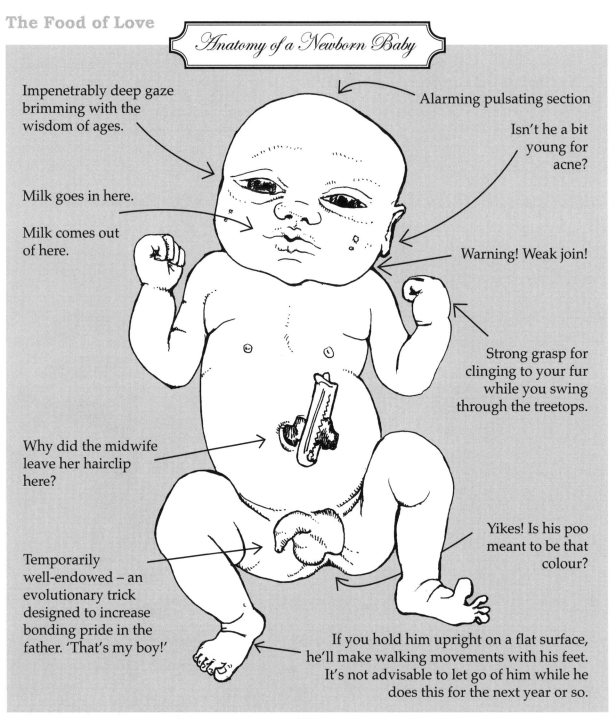

Impenetrably deep gaze brimming with the wisdom of ages.

Alarming pulsating section

Isn't he a bit young for acne?

Milk goes in here.

Milk comes out of here.

Warning! Weak join!

Strong grasp for clinging to your fur while you swing through the treetops.

Why did the midwife leave her hairclip here?

Temporarily well-endowed – an evolutionary trick designed to increase bonding pride in the father. 'That's my boy!'

Yikes! Is his poo meant to be that colour?

If you hold him upright on a flat surface, he'll make walking movements with his feet. It's not advisable to let go of him while he does this for the next year or so.

How to feed your baby

The thing is, babies don't feed from the breast the same way that they feed from a bottle.

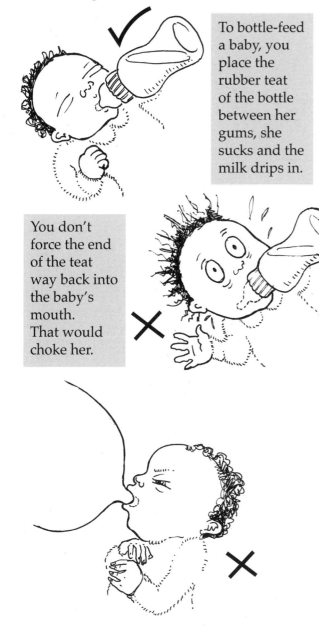

To bottle-feed a baby, you place the rubber teat of the bottle between her gums, she sucks and the milk drips in.

You don't force the end of the teat way back into the baby's mouth. That would choke her.

Breastfeeding is different. Here the baby's gums have to mash right up into the milk reservoirs, behind the areola (the dark bit), actually *in* the breast. The tongue pulses along the length of the breast, its rhythmic contractions help to keep the milk spurting, and the nipple itself is *right at the back of the baby's mouth*. The baby is described as being latched on. You'll see why. She gets hold of a sizeable portion of your breast, and she'll be pretty firmly attached. Don't get squeamish at the thought. It feels really nice.

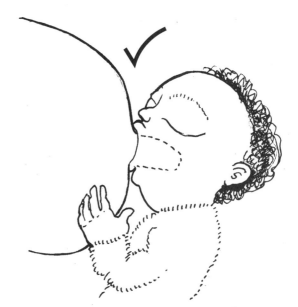

If your baby just sucks at your nipple, rather than your whole breast, breastfeeding is going to be an painful and unsatisfying experience for the two of you. Your baby won't get enough milk to satisfy her, and you will suffer from 'nipple trauma' (great phrase, huh?).

31

The Food of Love

You can see how this works for yourself. In late pregnancy, when you are enjoying a long, luxurious, uninterrupted bath (make the most of it!) try gently squeezing the area behind your nipples.

Make a C-shape with two fingers and thumb.

Push your hand back into your breast, towards your chest wall...

...gently roll your thumb over towards your nipple, and shift the pressure from your second to first finger.

Did you get a drop of milk? Did you? Wahey! Welcome to the world of lactation!

Don't worry if you can't find any milk. It will arrive when the baby does. Anyway, the point is milk is stored in a kind of 'well' deep inside the breast, behind the nipples. See if you can feel where it is. That's where the baby's mouth has to reach.

You don't need me to tell you that your nipples are extremely sensitive. The trick is to get that nipple right past your baby's gums and tongue, so they don't rub against it while feeding.

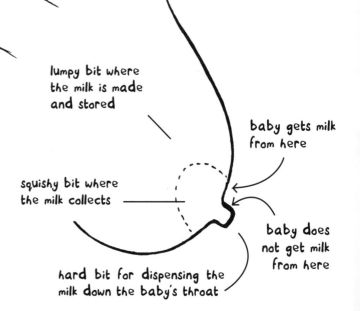

lumpy bit where the milk is made and stored

baby gets milk from here

squishy bit where the milk collects

baby does not get milk from here

hard bit for dispensing the milk down the baby's throat

Blimey. Here you are with a baby that's smaller than anybody you've ever met, and you have to feed her with breasts that are larger than any you've ever had before. It's not a good idea for someone else to try and force the baby onto your nipple, you have to do this yourself. To make it easier, here are some ridiculously detailed instructions.

1) OK, *relax*, you can do this. Tie your clothes out of the way so you can see what you are doing. Or take your top off. It is natural and good to hold your baby next to your skin.

Breastfeeding makes you thirsty so you will need a drink of water – sports bottles are good as you can knock them over as much as you like.

Your baby doesn't need to be screaming with hunger for you to feed her. Don't wait that long, or she'll learn she has to scream the house down every time she gets a bit peckish. When babies are hungry, they move their mouths sideways, and try to eat the edge of the blanket.

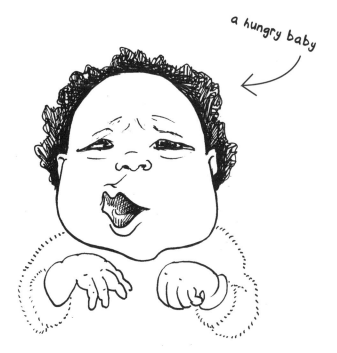

a hungry baby

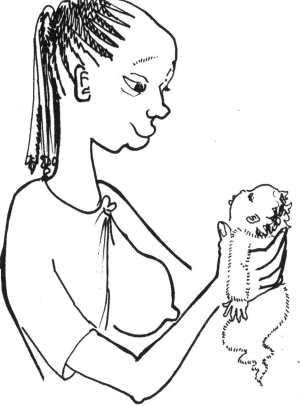

You have to be careful to **hold your baby in the right position** when you start out, because a newborn's mouth is so tiny, and you're both just learning how to do this. You may need pillows, and props, and special chairs, and a light or a torch at night. Hey, in a few months her mouth will have grown and you'll both be experts at this feeding thing. You'll be able to breastfeed while water-skiing by then.

33

2) *Sit up straight*. Have your thighs level, your feet resting flat on the floor (on some books if you need to), and your arms supported by firm arm rests or pillows. Have some more pillows handy to lay the baby on.

Don't hunch over your baby. It makes your breasts a funny shape and it will, in a very short space of time, give you a cracking backache.

If you're sitting on a sofa, try putting cushions behind you and underneath you so that you sit higher and straighter.

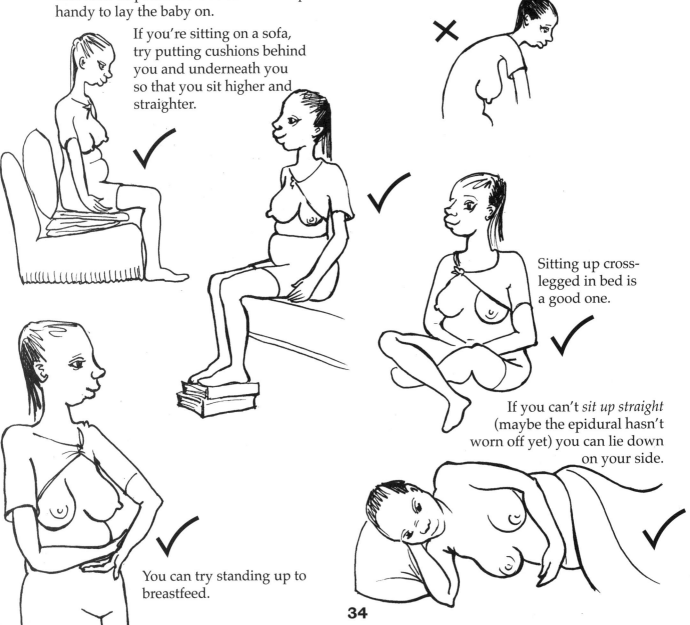

Sitting up cross-legged in bed is a good one.

If you can't *sit up straight* (maybe the epidural hasn't worn off yet) you can lie down on your side.

You can try standing up to breastfeed.

34

3) *Now get the baby.* There are a few different ways you can hold her...

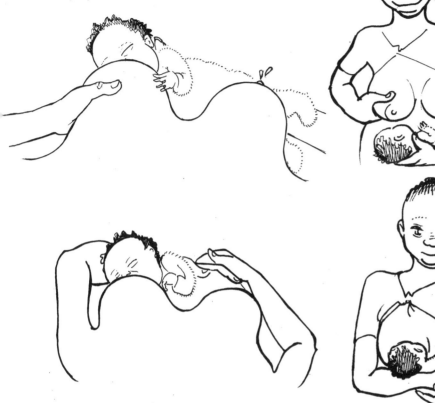

This is the **Transition hold**, and it's a very good one for beginners. You can support your breast and guide the nipple towards her mouth. Let her neck and the base of her head rest gently in the V between your finger and thumb. Don't cup the back of her head.

This is the **Cradle hold**. Slightly more tricky as you have less control. Support your baby's head on your forearm, not in the crook of your elbow (unless your nipples point out to the sides – some women's do).

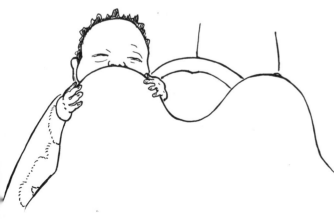

This is the **Rugby Ball hold**. Lay the baby under your armpit, again supporting her neck and shoulders, not her head. You can guide your breast with your free hand. This position is easy, comfy and useful because you have a hand free.

35

4) **Support the baby at the breast.** Stack up some pillows or folded blankets under the baby. Get a nice firm base so the pillows take her weight – that way your arms won't get tired during the feed.

If you are using the Rugby Ball hold, you may find that the arm of the chair or sofa will support the baby nicely. If you are lying down, play around with pillows and rolled up blankets – put them behind you and the baby so you don't roll away on the bed, or under either you or your baby until she's right at nipple height.

Don't stoop down or lean over your child. **Remember: bring the baby to the breast, not the other way round.**

Some women have high, perky nipples...

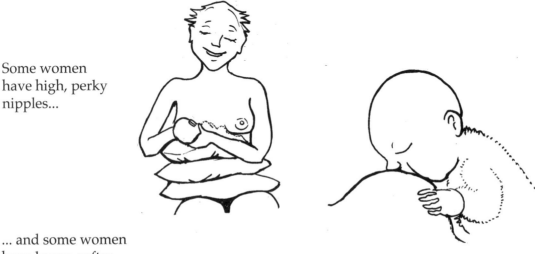

... and some women have lower, softer, larger breasts...

...therefore the number of pillows you need at this point is going to be a personal thing.

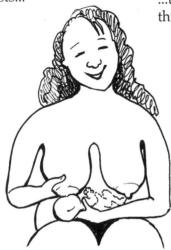

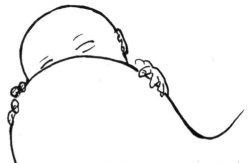

Where are your nipples? It's good to have a look in a mirror at some point and see.

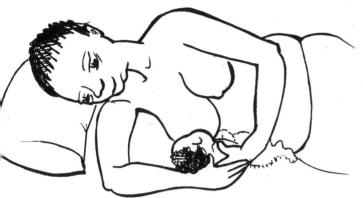

5) *Line her up, and tuck her body in close to you*. Rest her top lip by your nipple. Her head should be in line with her body, not turned to one side. It is hard to swallow when your head is turned to the side (try it). Let her naturally tip her head back a tiny bit to get her mouth and chin right up close to your breast.

6) *Nuzzle her into the areola, under the nipple.* See how clever she is? She already knows to root around and find the nipple. If she isn't interested, squirt a little milk on to her lips – that should remind her what this is all about.

7) *Wait* for the wide open mouth. See that tongue come out towards the nipple. Relax.

8) *Aim your nipple in towards the roof of her mouth*. Then, with the arm that's under the baby, bring the whole baby in towards you so she can get a nice big mouthful of breast. Did you get that? Bring the baby to the breast. Don't lean over and shove the breast into the baby.

Are her head and body still in a straight line? Her head doesn't want to be squashed forward to reach you.

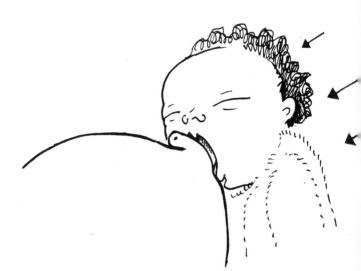

Or try this one: press your thumb into your breast so the nipple points up, away from her mouth, get her to take a big mouthful of the areola underneath your nipple, and *let your nipple fold upwards* as she sucks your breast into her mouth. This gets the nipple right to the back of her mouth, clear of the tongue.

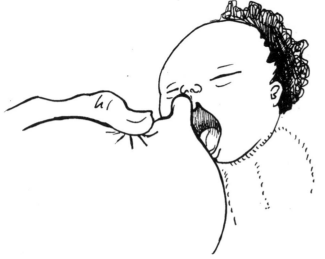

You can experiment with these two methods until you get her latched on right.

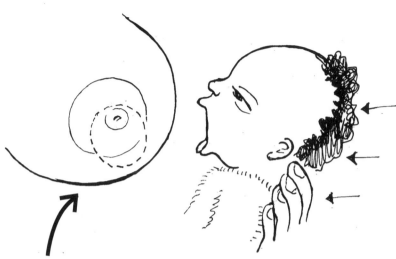

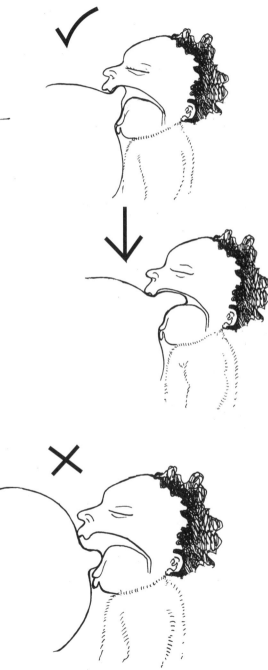

This is the target area. As you can see, you are actually trying to attach the baby a bit lopsided, with more of the underside of your breast in her mouth than the top.

Why? Well, there's a blinking great tongue in the middle of her mouth. If you try and poke your nipple into the centre of her mouth, it will get stuck on the tongue, instead of being sucked past it.

See what works best for your baby and your nipples. If you have large nipples and your baby has a small mouth, you'll probably have to try a few times. It's easier to attach a baby to nipples that are soft, so if your breasts are rock hard and full of milk, try squeezing some out onto a towel.

39

9) *How does it look?* It can be quite difficult to see when a baby is latched on properly, because her whole face is buried in your breast.

Her chin will be in close to your breast, and her bottom lip should be folded outwards. You can't see this unless you push a finger into your breast to check.

Keep her face level, so that both of her cheeks touch your breast equally. This is the most comfortable position for your nipples.

If you have large breasts then her nose may also be covered. Most babies can still breathe, through the little grooves at the base of their nostrils (I bet you never knew what they were for before). Some babies really can't breathe, so you need to gently *press the breast in* towards her to make an airway. You can also try snuggling her bottom in closer so that her nose tilts back away from the breast.

How does it feel? It should feel OK. Not painful. A bit intense maybe, but not sore.

She'll probably give a few deep sucks, then settle down to a pattern of sucking a few times, pausing for quite a few seconds, then sucking some more. Watch for the wiggling ears – that's a good sign that she's latched on well and getting some milk.

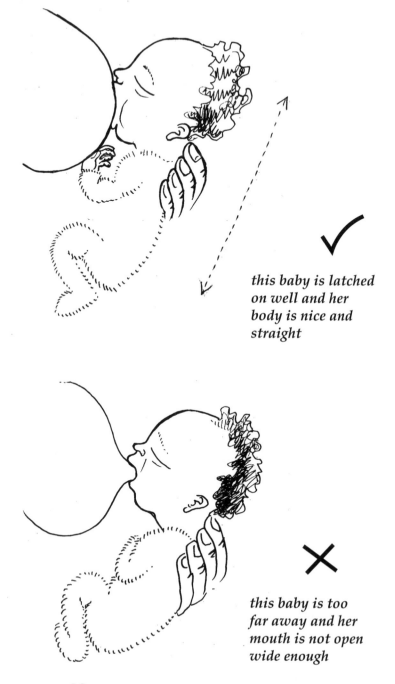

✔

this baby is latched on well and her body is nice and straight

✗

this baby is too far away and her mouth is not open wide enough

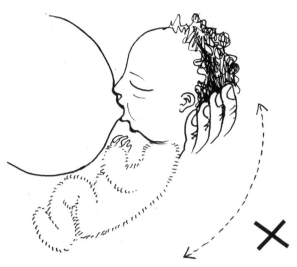

here the mother has flipped her baby's head forward – now she is at the wrong angle to suckle properly

If her mouth didn't open wide enough, then she'll just be sucking on the end of your nipple. It will feel like your nipple is being pinched or rubbed, which indeed it is. There will be space between her chin and your breast, and she will be pulled away from the areola rather than squashed onto it. Clicking or sucking noises are a sign that she may not be latched on right. Check that she hasn't sucked her bottom lip into her mouth.

If you haven't got her lined up with your nipple right, then your breast will be being dragged sideways into her mouth as she sucks. Ouch, more nipple trauma. If her head is bobbing about while she sucks, or if your breast is moving in little waves near her chin, then see how it feels to shift her slightly. When you get her lined up correctly then your breast and her head should both be fairly still, apart from the wiggling ears.

Not right? Break the suction by putting your little finger in the corner of her mouth.

Take her off

breathe out

relax, and try again.

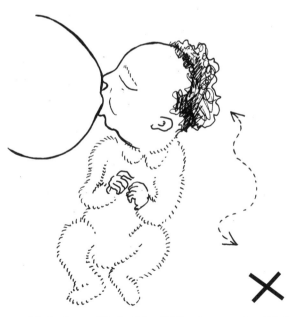

this baby will find it difficult to eat with her head and body twisted

Experiment a bit with how to get her on comfortably. No-one expects you to be able to do this right on the first go.

41

10) *What happens now?* Well, you just sit there and enjoy it. Suckling stimulates your brain to produce oxytocin (the same hormone that is produced when you make love – bonus!) which in turn makes your breasts contract, and squeezes out the milk.

This is known as the 'let-down reflex', which is spectacularly misnamed; you feel anything but 'let down'. It's also called the 'milk-ejection reflex'. I like the phrase 'milky feeling', because that's what it is.

A milky feeling differs from woman to woman. You might feel a warm glow of contentedness. You might feel a random patch of tingling, on your shoulder say, or in your toes. The feeling might be different depending on which breast is being suckled. You might not notice any particular feeling at all.

You will probably get thirsty when you breastfeed. Let's hope that water bottle is within reach.

You might feel some crampy period pains the first times you feed, as the oxytocin helps your womb shrink back to size. These 'afterpains' can be really bad with your second or third child. You can take paracetamol if you want to.

Your baby will relax and may look like she's asleep. If she actually does fall asleep she'll lose the latch and come off the breast. If this happens after only a few minutes then tickle her, talk to her, sit her up and see if she'll wake up to feed a little more.

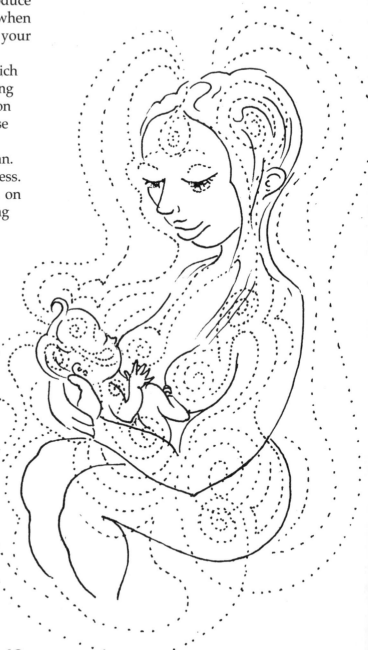

A scientific diagram of the let-down reflex

42

11) *Your baby knows when she's had enough.*
Your breasts fill up between feeds with watery fore-milk. This is a thin, sweet thirst-quencher. Your baby doesn't need bottles of water, as your body will cunningly make more of this in hot weather.

After a while, your breast feels deflated because this fore-milk has emptied out. *Don't take the baby off.* She hasn't had the good stuff yet.

The other two-thirds of the feed is produced *as you go along*. The baby slows down to a tranced out, blissful state where she munches a few times, then pauses for half a minute, then munches some more. This is when she's getting the cream. Your breast is forming rich hind-milk with all the energy in it for growing.

This is not comfort feeding. It is the building stuff of life. If you cut the feed short, stick a dummy in her mouth and get up to do something really urgent, then she'll probably drift off to sleep. But if you don't have to, then don't.

Letting your baby feed for as long as she wants to allows your body to learn how much milk she needs. This is the best way of programming your breasts to increase your milk supply.

Eventually she'll come off of her own accord with a snoozy, shiny 'milk-drunk' face.

It's lovely.

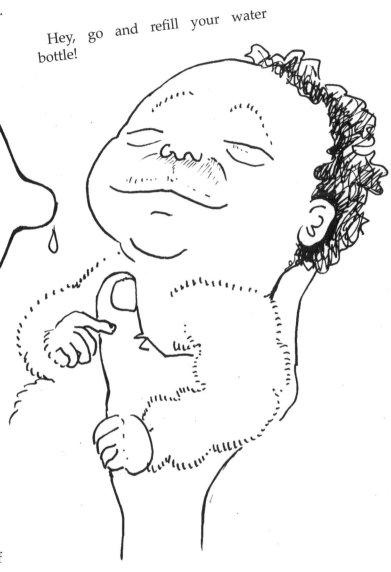

Hey, go and refill your water bottle!

12) *Hold her upright to see if any bubbles of wind come up.* See if she wants the other breast. She might do, or she might not.

13) *Feed from the other breast first next time.* There. That's how you feed a baby.

43

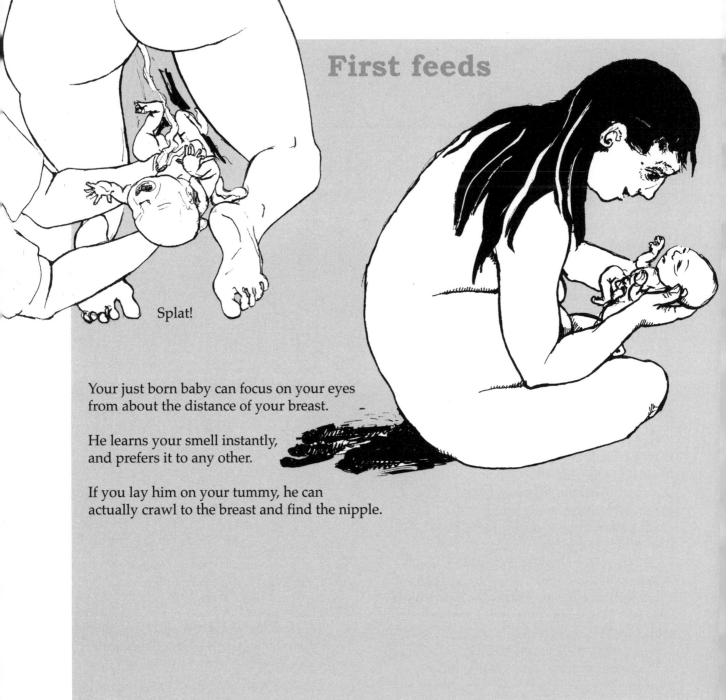

First feeds

Splat!

Your just born baby can focus on your eyes
from about the distance of your breast.

He learns your smell instantly,
and prefers it to any other.

If you lay him on your tummy, he can
actually crawl to the breast and find the nipple.

His first suckle helps your womb to contract
and expel the afterbirth.

The drops of milk that you give him are full of endorphins,
natural painkillers that ease his entry into the world.[1]

A baby can learn to feed in the first hour of his life...
given a chance.

My mother's experience

After my mother delivered her first baby flat on her back, handcuffed and shaved, with her legs strapped into stirrups, with a compulsory epidural which meant she couldn't feel the lower half of her body and a nurse had to tell her when to push (all standard practice in Montreal maternity wards in the 1970s)...

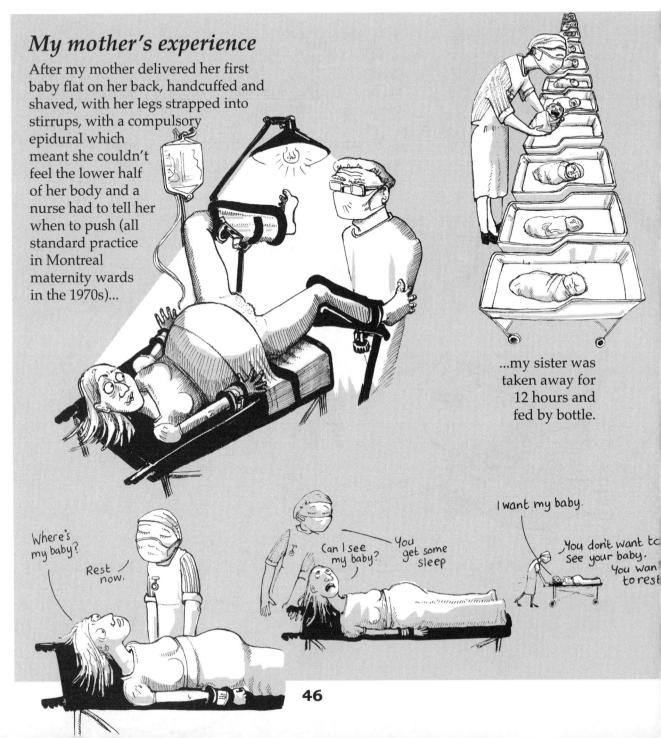

...my sister was taken away for 12 hours and fed by bottle.

Where's my baby?

Rest now.

Can I see my baby?

You get some sleep

I want my baby.

You don't want to see your baby. You want to rest

46

The following morning, having expressed a desire to breastfeed, my mum was reunited with her baby in a rather crowded room.

We've brought all the student nurses to watch breastfeeding because they won't get another chance.

Fortunately, Alice was a natural. Because a lot of babies forget, you know – the instinct is there right after birth but if you try for the first time the next day they don't know what to do. Not Alice.

The nurses said she'd had lessons in heaven, which was nice.

snuffle snuffle scoff scoff

47

My mother-in-law's experience

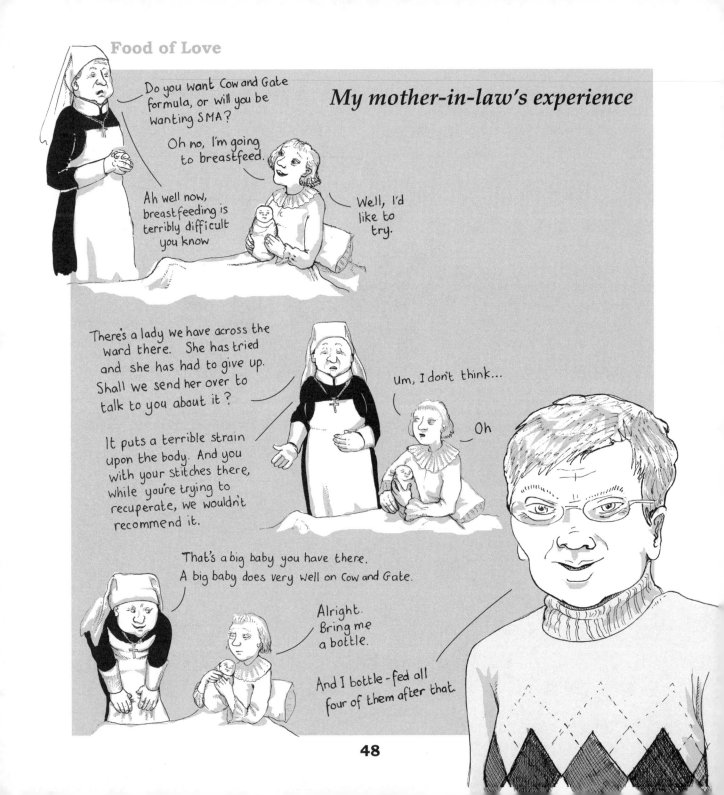

Do you want Cow and Gate formula, or will you be wanting SMA?

Oh no, I'm going to breastfeed.

Ah well now, breastfeeding is terribly difficult you know

Well, I'd like to try.

There's a lady we have across the ward there. She has tried and she has had to give up. Shall we send her over to talk to you about it?

It puts a terrible strain upon the body. And you with your stitches there, while you're trying to recuperate, we wouldn't recommend it.

Um, I don't think...

Oh

That's a big baby you have there. A big baby does very well on Cow and Gate.

Alright. Bring me a bottle.

And I bottle-fed all four of them after that.

48

Hospitals have improved a lot. The medical benefits of breastfeeding are now recognised and new mothers are told that breast is best. UNICEF instigated a Baby Friendly Hospital Initiative to integrate breastfeeding into hospital procedures which you can check that your hospital has adopted.

However, hospital staff can be incredibly overworked. You may find yourself in a situation which you haven't thought a lot about beforehand, with very little practical help. Stress actually inhibits your milk production, so this next section isn't designed to freak you out. Rather, it seems like a good idea to discuss some potential areas of difficulty ahead of time.

I mean, having a baby is a big deal. All the way through her first pregnancy, any sane, rational woman is going to be obsessed with wondering *how on earth a baby that large is going to come out of a hole that small*. This doesn't leave a great deal of time for wondering what you're going to do with the baby once it's here.

And here he is. And you've just found out why it is they call it labour. It's hard work. You may not have slept for days. That birth was exhausting. And now you have to learn a new skill, one you've not really seen done before. It might be fine. It might be easy. Or it might not.

You might have a drip in your arm, and a wound across your belly. You may find it difficult to sit up to breastfeed. Try feeding lying down. You might need help to arrange the baby.

Breastfeeding makes you thirsty. Chances are the hospital will provide you with half a plastic jug of tap water. It's not very appetising. Some fresh juice or mineral water is a good gift for a new mother.

You need to sleep in the same room as your baby, so you wake to feed him every time he needs it. That's the way your breasts learn to produce enough milk. It's ridiculous that there are still hospitals who cart newborn babies off to a nursery to sleep. It may be convenient for the hospital, but it doesn't help you and your bond with your child.

OK, so you're sleeping in the same room as your baby. There just happens to be another five women and their babies all asleep in the same ward, and now you don't want your baby to cry and wake them up. Remember, you are genetically programmed to respond to the sound of your own baby crying. It's not going to disturb anyone else as much as it upsets you. To them, it sounds like a baby crying. To you, it sounds like the end of the world.

Because when it comes down to it, if your baby is screaming, and you're not sure if he's feeding right, and all the staff seem too busy to check, at that point giving him a bottle of formula is going to seem like a very good idea. Ask for practical help to give him one good breastfeed. After that, he'll be happy, and you'll be more confident and things should be off to a good start. See if a sympathetic member of staff can sit with you to encourage you. You're not being demanding – it's important that your baby eats.

Right, check that your position, and the baby's position is good. Go back over everything in the previous chapter.

Tricky nipples...

Your midwife can refer you to a lactation consultant to help with breastfeeding difficulties. Here are some areas that could be of concern.

Nipple piercings shouldn't affect your breast-feeding experience as long as they are well healed. For this reason, don't get your nipples pierced when you are pregnant. You need to take your jewellery out while you feed and replace it afterwards. Pierced nipples might be more likely to leak milk, so invest in a lot of breast pads. Nipples that have been repeatedly pierced can be scarred, and could be more problematic.

Surgery on or through the breast can affect a woman's ability to produce milk. If you have had (or are considering) breast enlargement surgery, it is less problematic if the implant is placed beneath the pectoral muscle. If it is placed above it then it increases pressure on your milk ducts which doesn't help your milk supply.

Breast reduction surgery almost always results in some difficulties with milk production, because milk ducts and important nerves are severed. You are unlikely to be able to produce all the milk your baby needs, but you can still feed her what you've got. Milk ducts do reconnect with time, and your milk supply will get better with every pregnancy.

If you've had surgery, then see a lactation consultant so she can assess your progress. Keep your baby skin to skin. Use an electric breast pump after each feed to encourage your breasts to produce as much milk as possible, and don't be alarmed if you only get a few drops of milk at first. Be sure to wake your baby every four hours for feeds at night, and feed frequently during the day. Check her nappies to see if she's getting enough milk (see page 70). Massage your breasts during feeds and use breast compression (see page 71). Keep an eye on her weight gain. Your GP can prescribe domperidone to boost your supply, and there are herbs and foods that will help your milk production (look up 'herbal galactagogues' on www.kellymom.com and see page 71).

You may well need to supplement with formula, but this doesn't mean that you can't breastfeed. You can tape a thin tube to your nipple so your baby can drink formula while breastfeeding. Cunning! Ready-made nursing supplementers are manufactured by Medela or Lact-Aid, or you can make your own by taping a 0.6 feeding tube (ask the nurse) to your breast so the end sticks out fractionally further than your nipple. Put the other end in a cup of formula. There's a picture of a nursing supplementer on page 61.

The website www.bfar.org is an excellent resource which discusses all aspects of breast surgery and breastfeeding in detail.

Even though all breasts can produce milk, some women have *very little mammary tissue*[2]. There may be a link between this condition and polycystic ovarian syndrome. If you are very flat-chested, your breasts are widely spaced and tube-shaped, and *they didn't get larger during pregnancy* then see a lactation consultant about monitoring your milk supply. You can use the same measures as women who have had breast reduction surgery to breastfeed successfully.

Using nursing supplementers, massage and domperidone, even adoptive mothers can breastfeed. The process is known as *induced lactation*, and it's a lovely way to help an infant who has suffered trauma, separation or loss in his early life to be a baby again and to bond with his new mum[3]. Because adopted children have often been exposed to stress they are also vulnerable to infection and need the immunological protection that their adopted mother's milk can provide. Although some women are not able to produce breastmilk, many adoptive mothers manage to make some or eventually all of the milk their baby needs. What a result! Find detailed protocols for induced lactation on www.asklenore.info

Inverted nipples do not mean that you can't breastfeed. In fact, once you've established breastfeeding, you might well have nipples you can hang coat hangers off. It's just a little more tricky to get started.

Using special exercises or devices in pregnancy to treat inverted nipples doesn't usually make any difference, although if your husband doesn't mind applying a little gentle suction, that could be useful. Some nipples grow during pregnancy anyway. If yours still look flat once the baby arrives, gently squeeze the areola on either side of the nipple and see if you can encourage it to pop out. If you can, quick, latch the baby on. His incredible powers of suction will do the rest.

Some nipples retract further into the breast when you squeeze them. These are known as tethered nipples. Sandra Lang's book *Breast-feeding Special Care Babies*, which is probably the best book on breastfeeding that I've ever read, has the following recommendations:

• Spend lots of time cuddling your baby naked, or with just a nappy on (less messy) on your bare breasts.

• Don't worry if it takes time to get your breast-feeding started. You can express milk and feed your baby by cup (see page 59) in the meantime.

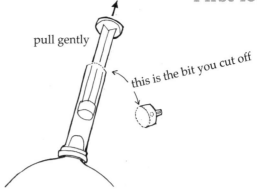

pull gently

this is the bit you cut off

• Cut the end off a syringe that is about the same width as your nipple. Pull the plunger out and put it back in the other end of the syringe. Place the rubbery end against your nipple, and very gently draw the plunger out one third of the way down the barrel. Only do this for a few seconds, and stop if it hurts. Push it back in to release the suction and see if this helps your nipple stick out.

• Lay your baby down and position your breast over him, make sure that his mouth is open wide and head tipped back slightly, then let your nipple fall into his mouth. He needs to get a big mouthful of the area under the nipple too. If you press gently on the areola just under his chin, it may encourage the nipple to come out.

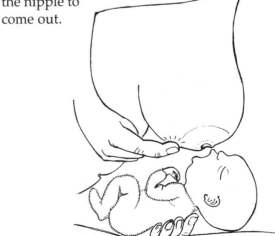

Tricky babies...

Some babies find it difficult to feed (and this applies to bottle-fed babies too).

If you were given pethidine or a general anaesthetic during labour, then your baby may be drowsy. This may last for up to a week. Wait four hours from the end of a breastfeed, and then wake her up and offer her the breast. She may be too little and weak to know that she's hungry. Keep her awake so she can feed a little longer. Undress her, play with her feet, blow gently on her face and talk to her – she will respond to the sound of your voice.

If she still keeps drifting off the breast then try switch feeding. Latch her onto the first breast for five minutes, then swap her over to the other breast for five minutes. Make sure you offer both breasts at least twice during the feed, so she gets to the fat-rich hind-milk. Also try breast compression (see page 71).

Stroke your finger down over your baby's nose and lips. She should stick her tongue out. She needs to be able to, to breastfeed well.

Very occasionally, a baby has difficulty suckling because her tongue doesn't protrude far enough over her lower gum to grasp the nipple well. Some babies' tongues are just really short. It's tricky to get them to latch on, then after a few minutes, they break the latch and may, annoyingly, fall asleep. Ten minutes later they need another microfeed. It's going to take some weeks for that tongue to grow, and you might get sore nipples in the meantime. Try the Dancer position on page 61 to see if it helps to keep the latch. It might be worth getting hold of a breast pump and expressing milk between feeds to keep up your supply. See if a lactation consultant can help you find a breastfeeding position that works well for you.

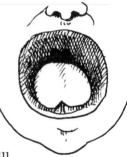

Sometimes the frenulum, the flap of skin under your baby's tongue, is too tight. This is known as a 'tongue-tie', and a classic sign is that her tongue will appear heart-shaped when she cries. Clipping the frenulum is a very minor surgical procedure which doesn't even need an anaesthetic. We're talking about a two millimetre cut here, equivalent to cutting a fingernail too short. She will be able to feed better immediately, and the sooner it is done, the easier it will be for her to learn to feed efficiently. Midwives used to keep a fingernail specially sharpened for the purpose apparently, but that was in the days before bottle-feeding became so fashionable.

A baby with a cleft lip can often press her lip up against your breast to seal it, and feed efficiently. Try the Dancer position (page 61) and lay your thumb over the cleft if she can't. Experiment with latching her on. A hissing noise is a sign that she hasn't quite got it right. Sometimes her latch will start out fine, and gradually slip off. Try again.

A cleft palate is more problematic. However, if you can get it to work, it is likely to be easier than bottle-feeding in the long run. Sometimes doctors are willing to fit a cleft obturator which may help. Squeeze a little milk out before you begin, so your nipples are nice and soft. Feed her propped upright against your belly, or sitting up in the Rugby Ball hold so the milk doesn't come back out of her nose. Her suck may be weak and inefficient, particularly if you can't see her ears wiggling. The Dancer position on page 61 will help a tired baby to breastfeed more easily. Feed her lots, express extra milk between feeds and check her nappies to see that she's getting enough milk (see page 70). A baby with cleft lip and palate will be prone to ear infections, so your milk is particularly good for her whatever way you end up feeding it to her.

'Why don't you feed him a bottle of formula, then you can see how much he's getting?'
Routine top-up feeds of formula are not a good idea for a tiny baby. Why? Look, the little thing has only just learned how to breathe, to smell, to taste and to see. Now you want him to learn how to feed. A rubber bottle teat is harder than a soft, mother's nipple, and you have to suck on it differently to get the milk out. Some babies who are initially fed with bottles find it difficult to learn how to breastfeed. This is known as 'nipple confusion' (another great phrase).

Plus your breasts have to learn how much milk to make. The more your baby suckles, the more they produce. And it works the other way round – if you feed your baby cows' milk, then next time you try to breastfeed your breasts are not going to be 'expecting' to produce enough milk to satisfy your baby. **Giving your baby top-up bottles is the quickest way to cause your milk supply to dwindle.**

But it is sometimes medically necessary to give a new baby some supplementary formula.

If your baby develops jaundice (yellow skin, dark eyes) on his first or second day of life, then he'll need a lot of fluid to help his liver work better. The jaundice may also make him drowsy. This is more common for babies delivered by ventouse suction. Formula top ups may be recommended or you can try expressing extra breast milk (see pages 56–59). Feed at least every three hours. Wait an hour after a feed, express as much milk as you can and put it in a sterilised syringe or bottle in the fridge. Before you next feed the baby, take the milk out of the fridge so it comes up to room temperature and give it to him after the feed as a top up. Switch feeding (see previous page) may also help him stay alert.

Jaundice that develops on day three or later is common and not usually problematic. Your doctor will probably advise that daylight and extra breastmilk are the cure. Feed him lots and put him in the window or take him outside. (Don't leave your baby in strong, direct sunlight as he may burn.) Your milk may take a while longer to get started after a Caesarean section, because it's a really big shock to the system. Don't worry, there's still colostrum there in your breasts, and every drop is precious for your baby. Frequent suckling will help it come on stream.

If part of your placenta was left in your womb, that can also depress your supply. Indications are offensive discharge and/or large blood clots.

If the midwives recommend supplementing with formula for a specific medical reason, then do it. Feeds don't have to be given by bottle. See the next section for details of feeding by cup or nursing supplementer. And don't stress. If you want to breastfeed, you'll still be able to.

Usually, your beautiful new baby doesn't need anything else except you. If you want to be sure that he's feeding enough, then bring him into your bed, lie him naked on your chest, cuddle him close and let him suckle all he wants to.

Which isn't very easy on a hospital ward.

Alice's first baby

This is my sister Alice's second most embarrassing experience of her life.

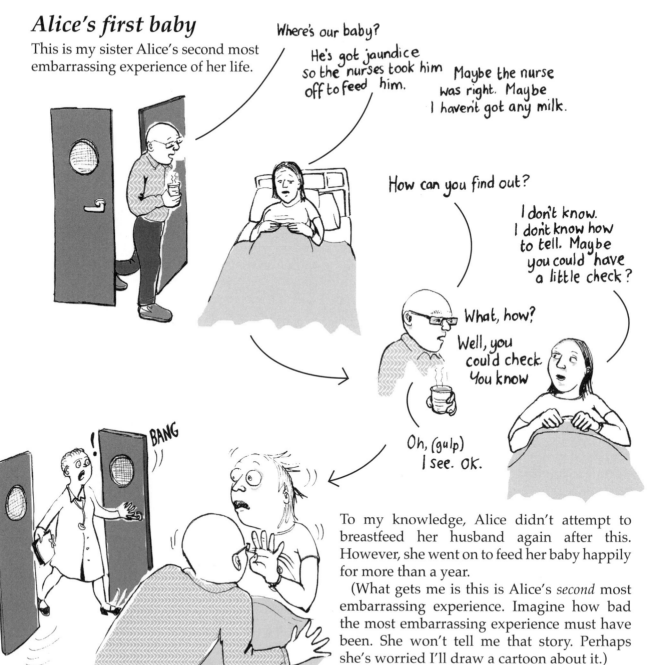

Where's our baby?

He's got jaundice so the nurses took him off to feed him.

Maybe the nurse was right. Maybe I haven't got any milk.

How can you find out?

I don't know. I don't know how to tell. Maybe you could have a little check?

What, how?

Well, you could check. You know

Oh, (gulp) I see. OK.

BANG

To my knowledge, Alice didn't attempt to breastfeed her husband again after this. However, she went on to feed her baby happily for more than a year.

(What gets me is this is Alice's *second* most embarrassing experience. Imagine how bad the most embarrassing experience must have been. She won't tell me that story. Perhaps she's worried I'll draw a cartoon about it.)

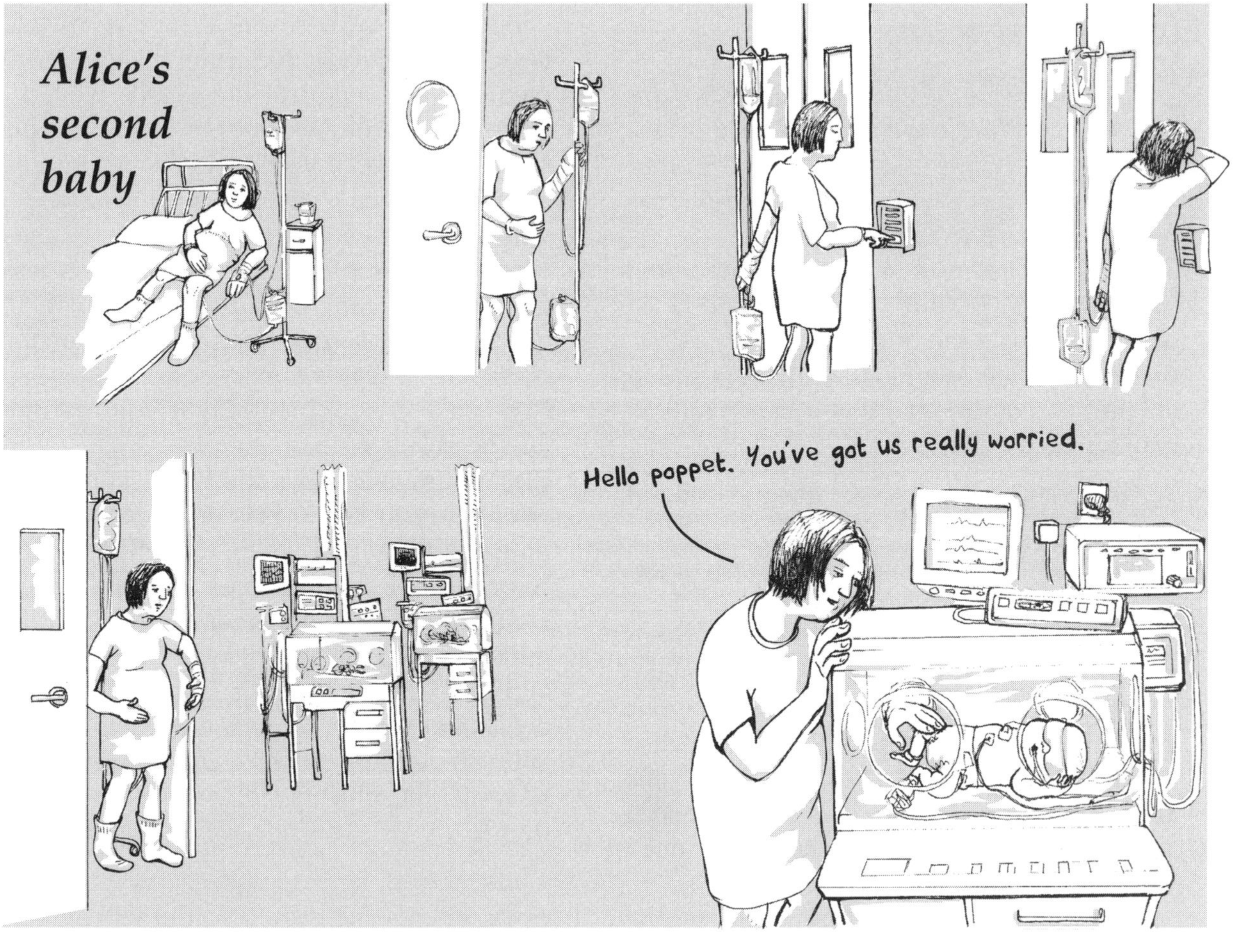
Alice's second baby
Hello poppet. You've got us really worried.

No-one expects their first experiences of breastfeeding to be in a neonatal intensive care unit. And while tiny baby medical care is amazing and life-saving, it's also very scary.

Now, unexpectedly, your baby isn't in your arms; he's in a box. If you're lucky, you can put your hands in to touch him, and then when you do, that heart monitor starts bleeping more quickly, so it feels like you've set off a burglar alarm. And the box is at chest height, so you can't even sit down while you look at him. In fact, to see him at all you have to press a buzzer and wait for ages to be let in. And then when you're there, what can you do?

Well, you can feed him. He needs your milk now, to nourish him and protect him from infection, and he needs it later, to help him grow healthy and smart. However, there are a couple of obvious obstacles in your way. Firstly, how do you get the milk out of you? And then, how do you get the milk into him?

Hand expression

My main source for the next six pages is Sandra Lang, author of *Breastfeeding Special Care Babies*. She has years of clinical practice. I, on the other hand, am a cartoonist. So many of these ideas are hers – I just drew the pictures.

If, for whatever reason, you are separated from your baby after birth, then it's a good idea to try to express some milk within the first six hours. Certainly try within the first 24 hours so your breasts get the idea that making milk is what they do. OK. How?

- Ideally you should be somewhere warm and reasonably private.
- Have a cuddle. Have a cry. Have a cup of tea. If you can, have a back massage.
- Anything that relaxes you, makes you laugh or reminds you of your baby is going to help with your milk production. So put your favourite music on your iPod, or watch a funny DVD. If you can't touch or see your baby, look at a photo of him and hold or sniff some of his clothes. Take some long, deep breaths and let the tension drop away.
- You'll have more milk first thing in the morning, so this is a good time to try.
- If it's evening, turn down the lights. Candlelight is nice. Light a room burner with some essential oils if that helps you to relax.
- For the first few days after the birth you will produce colostrum – drops of thick yellow or clear liquid. There isn't very much of this. A healthy newborn who is feeding well will only take between one and 10 ml at a feed – that's two teaspoons full at the most. The easiest way to collect colostrum is for a reassuring person to sit with you and suck it up into a sterile syringe. Colostrum is wonderful medicine, so every drop is precious.
- After a couple of days your milk will become more milky. You'll need a sterile container to squirt it into, and a towel in case you miss.
- Wash your hands and fingernails.
- Massage your breasts. Lean forwards and gently shake them. Knead them, stroke them or even tickle them, always moving from the outside, in towards your nipple.
- Play with your nipples. Maybe your partner will be able to help.
- Cup your breast in your hand, and move your fingers in towards your nipple. Feel the lumpy fibrous area where the milk is made. Now feel the squishy part where the milk well is. Rest your fingers at the edge of the milk well and squeeze gently. Push right in and back. Don't let your fingers slide over the skin and don't scrunch the skin up.
- You can also try pushing your fingers back towards the chest wall, and rolling your thumb towards the nipple. See page 32.

The first few times you squeeze nothing will happen. Then some drops of milk will appear. Eventually you should be able to get some squirts of milk. Squirt, pause, squirt, pause, squirt, until the flow reduces back to drops. Then rotate your hands around the breast and repeat the process. Do this right round the breast so that you drain all the lobes. Page 161 tells you how to store breastmilk.

If you're really not getting anything, try more relaxation measures. A warm bath or shower can be a good place to try again. Experimentation and gentle persistence will eventually pay off.

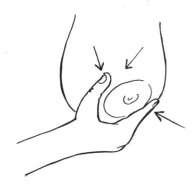

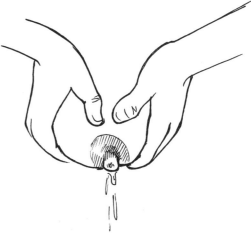

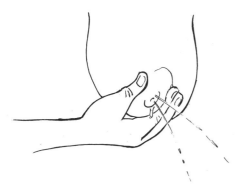

*one-handed and
two-handed techniques*

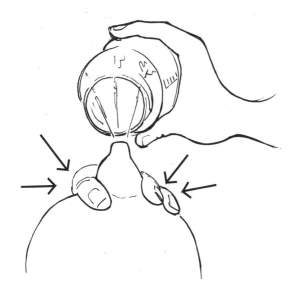

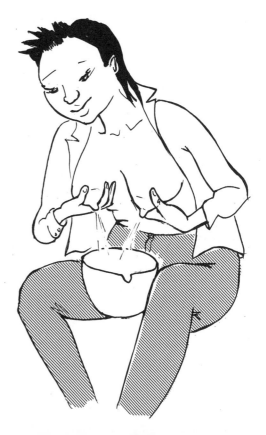

57

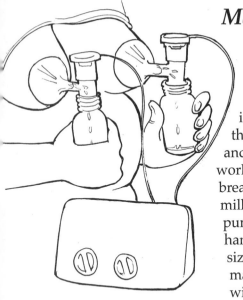

Mechanical expression

The beauty of hand expression is that you can find the places, rhythms and techniques that work best for your breasts and for your milk flow. Mechanical pumps, on the other hand, come in one size, which may or may not work well with your size breast. If you have the chance to try different pumps then do. If they come with silicone inserts, see whether they work better if you take them out. Be gentle when you pump – it is possible to damage your nipples if you're too enthusiastic. Your nipples look very strange when you pump.

Having said that, using a hospital-grade electric pump on both breasts simultaneously is the most efficient way to build up and maintain your milk supply. Sterilise the pump and collection containers before you begin and wash your hands. Massage your breasts, and use the relaxation techniques from page 71. Start on the lowest setting and gradually increase the suction. It may help to pause a few times during a session, and shift the funnel around your nipple slightly so all the lobes of your breast are stimulated. Try not to think about cows!

Professional electric pumps are brilliant. If you have to use one for a while, try cutting some slits in the front of your bra to hold it in place – then you get your hands free. The only down sides are that they are expensive, bulky, and may need servicing to work properly.

Hand expression can be the next most efficient method once you've mastered your technique. This is the cleanest, simplest and most portable way to express milk. Hand-expressed milk contains higher levels of natural sodium, which is good for your baby, particularly if he is premature. After you have finished on an electric pump, see if you can hand-express a little more.

Hand pumps may also work well for you. They can be ridiculously complicated to assemble and they are not as efficient as a hospital pump, but they are much cheaper and you can take them anywhere. Cheap commercial electric pumps are really only hand pumps with a noisy motor on them, with no real advantage over the manual version.

Clean and sterilise all parts of the pump and collection bottle before each use. Only ever use a pump which is marketed as appropriate for use for expressing milk for baby feeding. Other mechanical methods of milk collection are not sterile and are unsafe.

How often and how much

You can express all the milk your baby needs, as long as you get enough rest and support so you can spend enough time doing it. Even if formula is recommended, mixing it with your breastmilk will make it easier for him to digest, and will give his immune system a boost.

You will need to express milk eight times every 24 hours if you are not breastfeeding yet. Do it first thing in the morning, and last thing before you go to bed. Wake up at night to express as well, because your prolactin levels are higher at night. Try not to go more than seven hours without expressing.

It is quite common for your milk supply to drop after you have been expressing well for some weeks. Stay in bed all day, increase the number of times you express and see if any of the tips on page 71 will help.

Don't time your expressions; just do it until you're not getting any more milk. At first you'll only be able to do a few minutes on each side. Build up to more than ten minutes on each breast. If it regularly takes you more than an hour then see if an expert can help you improve the efficiency of your technique, and also check that the pump is working properly. But you are providing optimum nutrition and immunological protection for a tiny vulnerable human being. As you can see, this is a full-time job.

How to stop

Once your baby is breastfeeding successfully, you will need to gradually reduce the amount that you pump over a period of five days. Use a hand pump. Express milk three times a day,

before you feed your baby so he gets your good, fatty hind-milk. Express a little less every day.

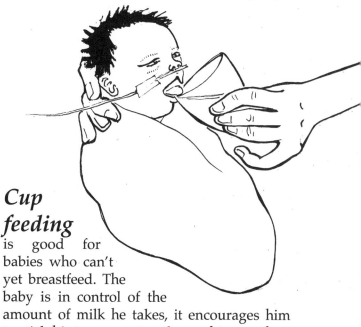

Cup feeding

is good for babies who can't yet breastfeed. The baby is in control of the amount of milk he takes, it encourages him to stick his tongue out and open his mouth to feed, and helps him co-ordinate his sucking and swallowing reflexes.

• Swaddle your baby so his arms are wrapped up down by his sides, and put a bib under his chin. Cuddle him fairly upright in your arms.

• Hold a little cup of breastmilk very gently against his mouth so that the milk is just level with his lips. You can use a sterilised egg cup, or the plastic cap from a feeding bottle if it has a smooth rim.

• He can then lap the milk into his mouth like a little kitten. Older premature babies learn to sip the milk. *Don't tip the milk into your baby's mouth* – let him take it himself.

• Milk can also be spoon-fed to a tiny baby using the same method.

Kangaroo care

Once your baby is stable enough to be moved from the incubator he can start to have his first comfort at the breast. It doesn't matter whether he is still too little to breastfeed, just being held in your arms is beneficial. This is known as kangaroo care. Dads can do it too. One amazing thing about kangaroo care is that it allows us to see scientific evidence of the benefits of loving human touch.

Babies who are cared for by kangaroo care are calmer, warmer, sleep better, have more stable heart rates and breathing, a lower risk of disease and infection, are less stressed, experience less pain, may grow better, definitely feed better, develop better and go home sooner than babies in incubators[4].

A baby who is unable to breastfeed can suck, lick or nuzzle close to the nipple. You can drip milk from a syringe into his mouth while holding him like this, or express milk directly onto his lips. Once your breastfeeding starts to become established, don't be discouraged if he feeds well one day but is unable to the next. Childhood development is like that.

Check with the nursing staff that they won't give your baby dummies or bottles: there is a real chance that they will interfere with his ability to latch onto the breast. Expressing milk to feed a baby who will only take a bottle traps you into an exhausting situation which can require weeks of perseverance to remedy.

If your baby does become used to artificial teats and rejects the breast, try stimulating your nipple so that it is hard and pointing it up towards the roof of his mouth when you latch him on. Nipple shields might help.

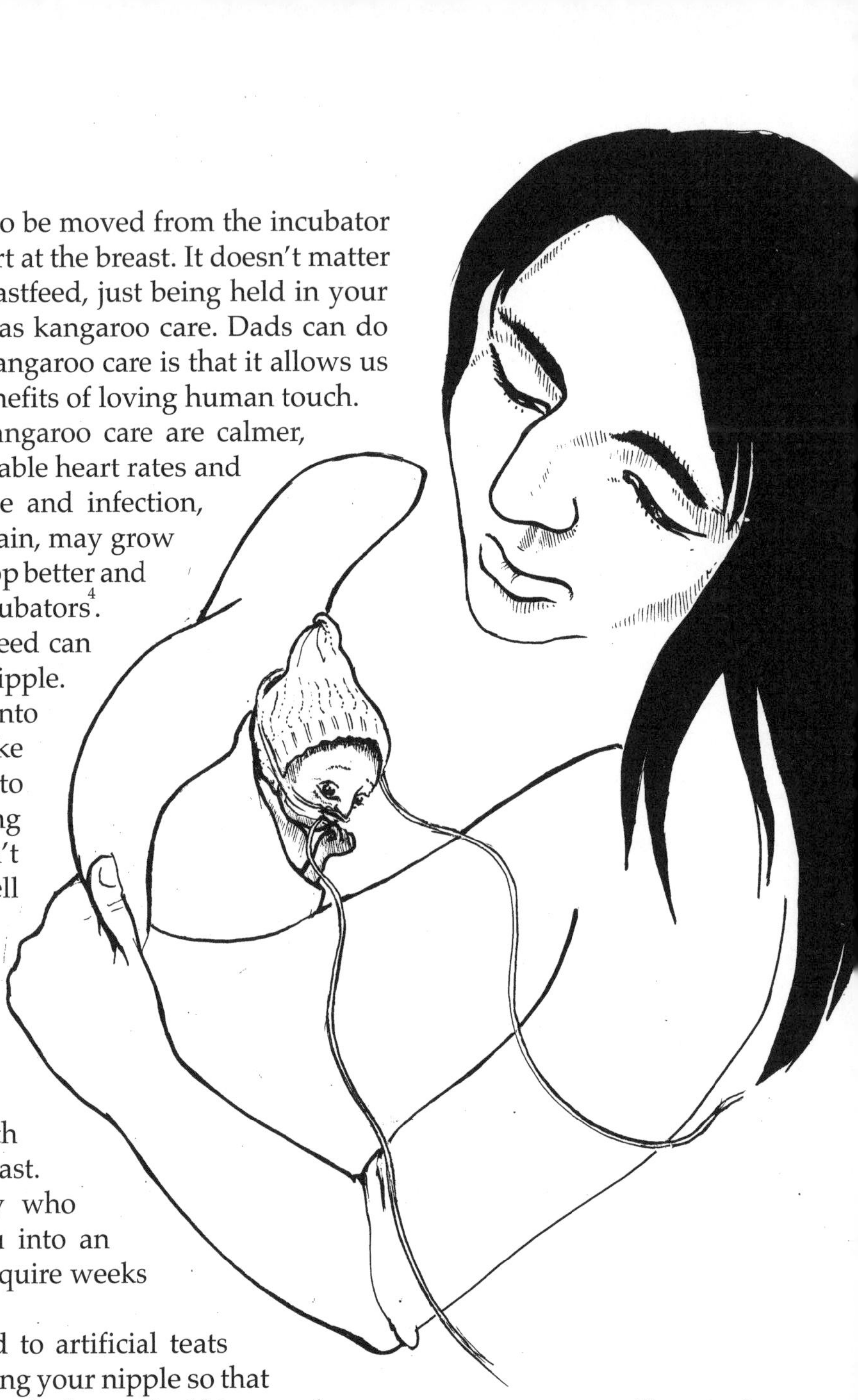

Keep trying.
Babies can surprise you.

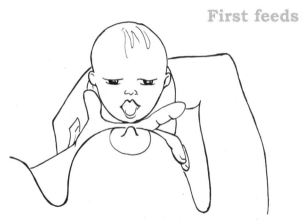

This is the **Dancer position**, and it's a good one to use to help a baby to feed if they are very weak or have problems attaching to the breast.

- Sit the baby upright at the breast.
- Cup your breast with the palm of your hand and let your index finger and thumb wrap around your baby's chin. Help her to maintain her attachment like this throughout the feed.

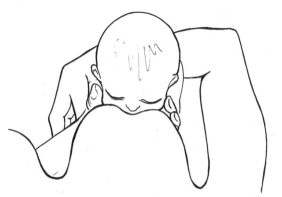

Here's a **nursing supplementer** in action, which can be used when your baby is too weak to suckle effectively, or if you have trouble with your milk supply (see pages 50–51).

- If you have to use one on a regular basis, you'll need three: two to be kept in the fridge full of milk, and one hung round your neck to come up to body temperature.
- You can wean a baby off it by gradually taping the tube further away from your nipple.

61

A home birth

That was... ...long.

This is me and Kate and Pete and their very new baby. Now we all know that the first hour of life is a good time to put the baby to the breast. But Kate has just been through 55 (count 'em!) hours of labour. The good thing about her home birth with an independent midwife is that no-one was standing over her with a stopwatch threatening to put her on a drip if she didn't produce a baby by the end of their shift....

Omigod! Well done!

Well done all three of you!

I just trod on something squishy.

...and now no-one's going to chivvy her along with the ultimatum 'We need to see you breastfeed before you leave the delivery room.'

Everyone's taking a moment to catch their breath.

They all got in the birthing pool, where the baby had her first feed.

It was quite a long feed.

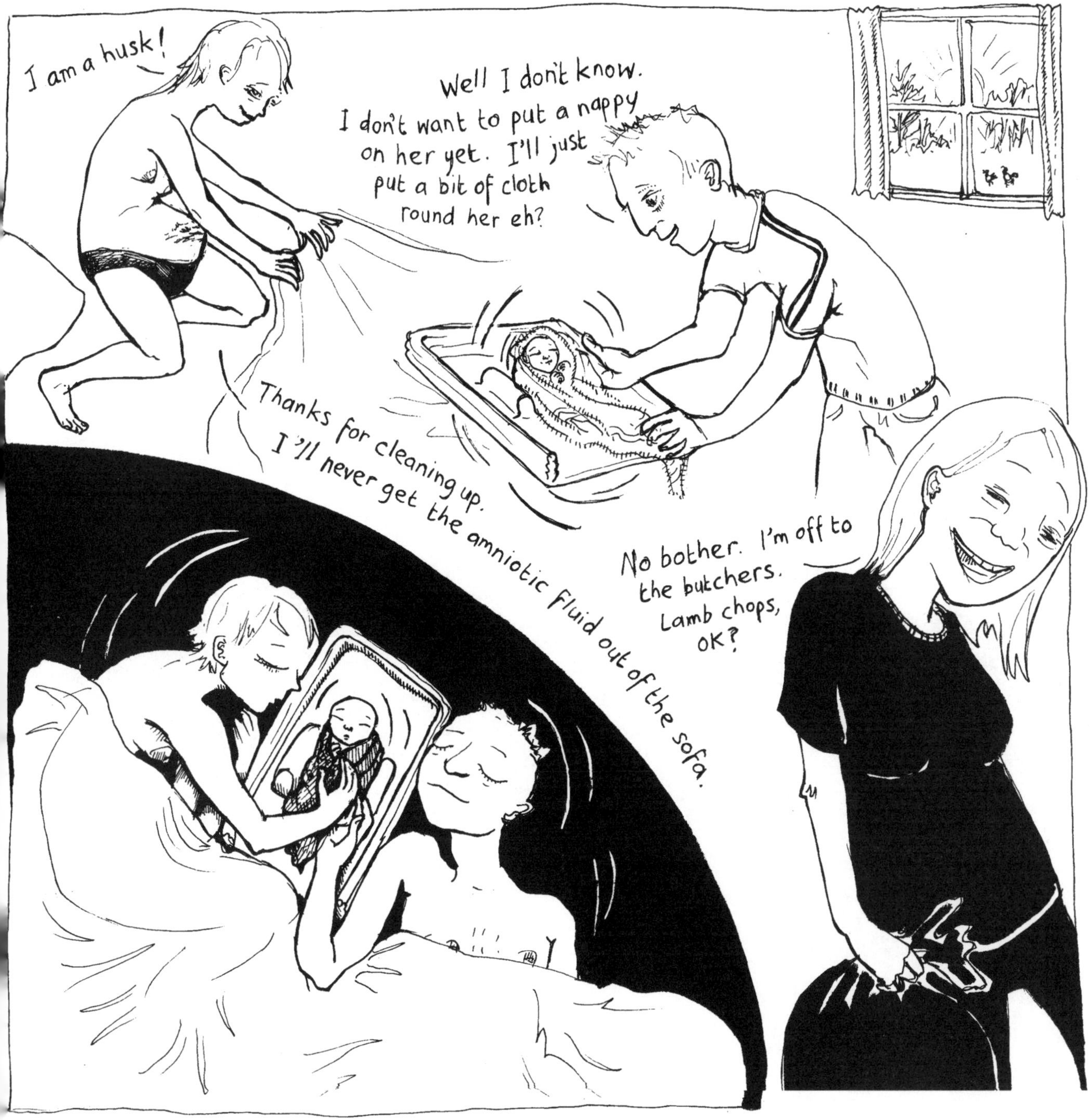
I am a husk!
Well I don't know. I don't want to put a nappy on her yet. I'll just put a bit of cloth round her eh?
Thanks for cleaning up. I'll never get the amniotic fluid out of the sofa.
No bother. I'm off to the butchers. Lamb chops, OK?

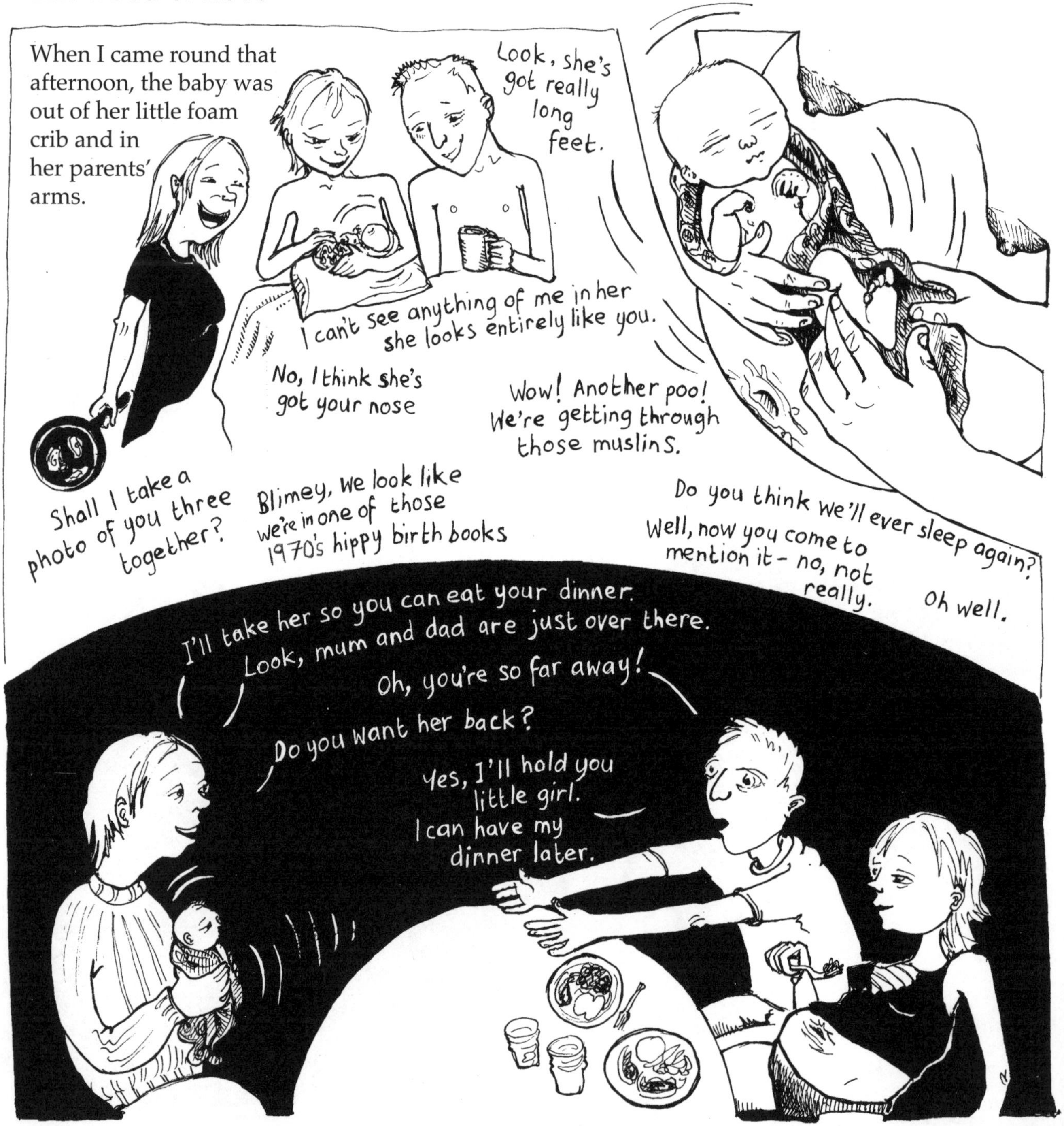
When I came round that afternoon, the baby was out of her little foam crib and in her parents' arms.
Look, she's got really long feet.
I can't see anything of me in her she looks entirely like you.
No, I think she's got your nose
Shall I take a photo of you three together?
Blimey, we look like we're in one of those 1970's hippy birth books
Wow! Another poo! We're getting through those muslins.
Do you think we'll ever sleep again?
Well, now you come to mention it - no, not really.
Oh well.
I'll take her so you can eat your dinner.
Look, mum and dad are just over there.
Oh, you're so far away!
Do you want her back?
Yes, I'll hold you little girl.
I can have my dinner later.

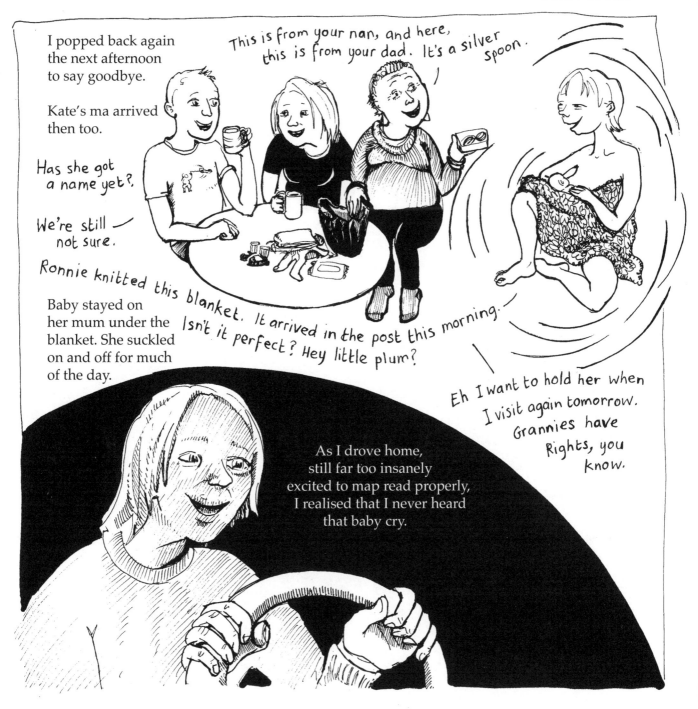

I popped back again the next afternoon to say goodbye.

Kate's ma arrived then too.

This is from your nan, and here, this is from your dad. It's a silver spoon.

Has she got a name yet?

We're still not sure.

Ronnie knitted this blanket. It arrived in the post this morning. Isn't it perfect? Hey little plum?

Baby stayed on her mum under the blanket. She suckled on and off for much of the day.

Eh I want to hold her when I visit again tomorrow. Grannies have Rights, you know.

As I drove home, still far too insanely excited to map read properly, I realised that I never heard that baby cry.

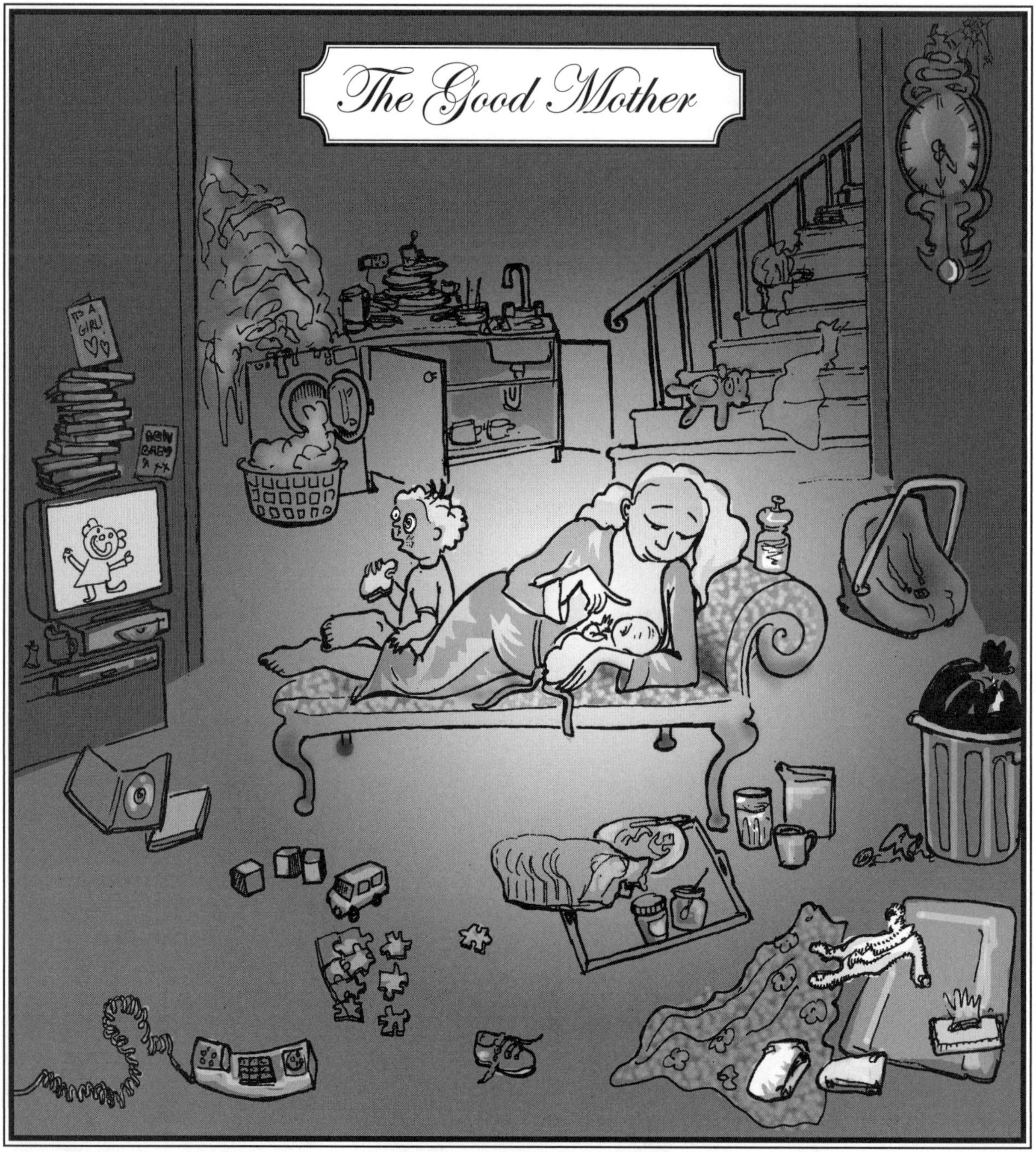
The Good Mother
IT'S A GIRL!

New mother care

Get some rest.

The period after your baby is born is traditionally known as your confinement; six weeks of staying in and focusing on your and your new baby's needs. Six weeks. Got it? Clear your diary. Even if you feel fine, rest completely so you can heal completely.

This is going to take some arranging. In the old days, neighbours or family members would turn up when a woman had a baby and take over the domestic chores. Nowadays, very few women can rely on this kind of automatic support. And after the birth you feel raw and emotional: fear of rejection can prevent you from asking for help.

Consider this though. Have you ever done a 24-hour-a-day job before? Where you have to wake up every two hours? Without a break. Or any days off. And did you start this job immediately after undergoing a painful, major medical procedure? Where you may have lost a lot of blood and/or been injected with strong prescription drugs. AND did this job involve a major, irreversible change in your role in life, with serious emotional ramifications (most of them good)?

In this situation, you're going to find it difficult to cook, wash up and hang the laundry out.

If you have a partner, arrange between yourselves that they can take over completely on the domestic front. That may not be as easy as it sounds. Feminism is meant to have won us equality with men over the last 30 years. In fact, for many women it has meant that we now hold down full-time jobs, like men, but also undertake pretty much all the housekeeping and childcare. Unconsciously, that may be what you and your partner are expecting you to do. That's a ridiculous expectation, which is going to mean your baby will suffer.

If you don't have a partner, do you have a good friend or relative who can come and look after you? It may be worth going to stay with relatives, although you'll need to co-ordinate that with your midwives so you still get some antenatal care. My single-mother-with-twins friend had a rota so someone came round every single day. That's a good idea.

If you have other children, consider getting someone to come and keep them occupied. Again, this is easier said than done. You're probably worrying that they'll be jealous of the new baby. Yes, they almost certainly will. But that doesn't mean you should overtax yourself trying to be supermum. Remember how it's generally easier to look after two children happily playing, than it is to keep one occupied? Ask your children's friends' parents for some major babysitting favours, and then pay them back in six months' time.

Let the housekeeping go. It doesn't matter. Your baby does. I tend to find the phrase 'A clean house is a sign of a wasted life' useful at such times. I have a mug with it on, which brings me much solace.

Ask visitors to bring cooked meals with them. Keep visits short, or rope people into doing things for you. You've provided the baby who they have come to see, now they can make the tea. Why not leave them with the baby for a bit while you *get some rest*?

Don't tidy up for visits from the health visitor. She only wants to see that your baby is happy, not that the carpet is clean. My friend's health visitor ticked her off for cleaning up, and told her that she wanted to see some dirty dishes in the sink at the next visit.

Make sure you eat and drink enough. If you notice your urine is dark then drink extra fluid. There's more about diet on pages 78–81.

If you don't usually nap in the daytime, then learn. It's a vital skill for early years survival.

None of this is going to happen unless you accept that it needs to. You are going to spend some time finding out about motherhood. Pregnancy was not a temporary hiatus in your usual routine. You can't just pop a baby out and expect to pick up everything where you left off. Your baby needs you. He's really important. Drop everything else, relax, and enjoy him.

Here are some more tips for post-birth healing:
- Take the sting out of going for a wee by pouring some warm water with a few drops of lavender essential oil in over yourself.
- Also try the homeopathic remedy Hypericum for shooting pains in your bits, Bellis Perennis for deep bruising pain, and Staphyisagria for any birth event that feels like you were invaded. Either homeopathy works (which it seems to) so it will help, or you've eaten a small sugar pill which isn't going to do you any harm.
- Eat regular healthy food. See page 78.
- Keep yourself warm, especially round your middle. Hot water bottles are good.
- If you're feeling really wiped out and having difficulty recovering, acupuncture can help.

Hey, you! If you're reading this book and you're not just about to have a baby then go and make dinner for someone who just has!

Have I got enough milk?

Yes. Regardless of the size or appearance of your breasts, they never run out of milk. They sometimes look and feel deflated, but if you squeeze them, you'll see that there's always a drop there. As long as you're getting enough *time* to feed your baby, and enough *rest* after the birth to care for her, then your breasts are going to work fine.

Think about it; any mammal who couldn't produce enough milk for her offspring would have been a genetic non-starter and become extinct long ago.

But, I'm not going to lie to you here, small babies feed a *lot*.

When my son was about six weeks old, there came a day when I realised I was knackered, and I stayed in bed with him all day. Now I can't be sure of this, because I was asleep for some of the time, but I think he fed solidly for *six hours*. I never read anything like that in any of the books. I was so hungry when I got up!

A tiny baby's mouth is small, so she milks the breast slowly, and her stomach is small (about the size of her fist) so it empties out quickly. So a young baby does a lot of suckling. After a few months, she will become more efficient at feeding, so stick at it. Also, once you've done three months of good breastfeeding, you can be sure that your milk supply is good. At that point, if you want to, you can start cheating and using dummies or the odd bottle of formula, without your supply diminishing (see page 180).

So many women these days lose confidence in their breastfeeding because they think their milk isn't satisfying enough. It's just not true – that's how often small babies eat. If your baby feeds happily, and comes off the breast when she's full, and breastfeeding is painless and unrestricted, things are going well.

If your baby cries and fights the breast, then falls asleep after a few sucks, then you need help to improve your attachment. Sometimes, just a small adjustment can make all the difference.

Babies grow incredibly quickly in their first year of life. Watch out for growth spurts, which may happen at about three weeks, six weeks and at twelve weeks (or at any other time!). These are the *you can't be hungry already because I just fed you* times. Your baby might need to feed all day, and your breasts may feel like there's nothing there. There is, remember.

Say your baby has been feeding almost constantly for days, and you decide to give her a bottle of formula. Watch as she guzzles it straight down, instantly falls asleep, and isn't hungry for another four hours. *This doesn't mean that you haven't got enough milk.* All this proves is that reconstituted cows' gloop is difficult for your baby to digest. Formula milk sits like stodge in your baby's gut and her body has to work hard to digest it. Breastmilk, on the other hand, being the perfect food, can be completely digested in twenty minutes.

Growth spurts are a good time to shelve new projects and spend the day being connected with your baby. Take a bath with your baby, or spend some time in bed with her. The renewed closeness will encourage your breasts to increase your milk supply. If this isn't possible, a good baby sling will allow you to feed your baby on the move. (See page 158.)

But how do I know she's getting enough milk?

It's normal to worry about everything to do with caring for your baby. Is she sleeping at the right times? Is she too hungry? Why isn't she smiling / crawling / walking / speaking / passing her GCSEs yet? This process of continually evaluating whether your baby is OK, and whether your mothering is OK, is what makes you a good parent. It keeps you alert to any little sign that your baby does need help, and it helps you know your baby better than anyone else in the world.

If your baby is waking up to feed, then she's getting enough milk. A baby that isn't eating enough is sleepy and reluctant to feed, even after four or five hours' sleep. Try switch feeding (page 52) if she is dozy.

Other early signs of dehydration in a newborn baby are a dry mouth (check with your finger) and a sunken fontanelle. This is the soft bit on the top of the baby's head. It should be flat. If it sinks in, then she needs extra fluid.

Four to six squidgy disposable nappies, or six to eight soggy cloth nappies in 24 hours, is a good indication that feeding is going well.

Keep an eye on her poos in the early days. You want to see a black, tarry poo on the first or second day. By day three the colour should start to change and by day five it should be soft and yellow. If your baby is still passing black poos on day four or five, she isn't getting enough milk. If her poos tend to be greenish and liquid she may be getting too much fore-milk and not enough hind-milk. Ask for help with your breastfeeding technique.

Weight gain

Nearly all babies lose some weight in the first week of life. After that your baby should start gaining, and his weight will be plotted on a growth chart. These charts are based on the average of all babies in your country in recent years. It is worth remembering that the majority of babies in the UK are currently fed formula, and these babies are fatter and heavier than breastfed babies. And this means that the majority of breastfed babies are going to look below average on the weight charts. Which can knock your confidence a bit.

If you know that you're feeding your baby a lot, yet he keeps slipping down a curve on the weight growth charts, there is a possibility that he could be allergic to food substances that are passing into your breastmilk (see page 81). If he does, he is likely to show other signs of an allergic reaction. Or he might just be a whippet. Maybe his dad is skinny too.

The following measures to increase your milk supply may also help.

Do you really have *low milk supply*? Breasts often stop feeling full when a baby reaches five or six weeks of age. That's an indication that they have become super-efficient at making milk. You can't tell how much milk your baby is getting by looking at your breasts.

Make sure your baby is latched on well. Getting your breastfeeding technique assessed by a professional lactation consultant or breastfeeding counsellor will improve your confidence.

Don't cut your baby's feeds short – wait for him to come off on his own. Feed your baby whenever he seems interested. Frequent feeds will increase your milk supply, because stimulating your nipples lots will help your prolactin (breastmilk hormone) production, and because when your breasts get full, they get the message to slow down milk production.

Massaging your breasts before you feed can encourage the milk to let down quicker. Relaxation measures such as getting a back-rub or a cuddle from your partner can also help. Lighting soothing essential oils or having a warm bath or shower are also good.

Try *breast compression*. Hold your breast with your free hand during a feed, with your fingers underneath and your thumb on top. Watch your baby feeding. At first he should take long gulps at the breast, opening his mouth wide for a moment, pausing, then closing it again. After a while he will settle down into something that is more like nibbling or fluttering. At this point squeeze your whole breast with your hand and release (don't do it so hard that it hurts). This pumps the milk down towards your nipple. The baby should switch back to the more active form of feeding. Keep this up throughout the feed.

Express extra milk using a hospital-grade electric pump, or by hand (see pages 56–58). It is normal to get very little milk the first few times you pump, but you should find that if you keep trying three times a day for a week, the amount that you get each day will increase. This extra stimulation will help build up your milk supply.

If you are very concerned about your baby's weight or milk intake you can feed the expressed milk to him by cup or by bottle after a feed. (Don't do this for weeks on end, or the baby will learn to prefer the bottle, which is slightly easier to feed from, to the breast.) Otherwise simply freeze it for future use (see page 161).

Lay off alcohol and cannabis. If you smoke, then give up or cut down. Eat regular, nutritious meals (see page 78). There is no evidence that exercise harms your milk supply.

Oestrogen-based hormonal contraceptives such as the Pill can commonly interfere with your milk supply. Choose another form of contraception (see pages 172–173).

Drink fenugreek herbal tea: make a strong brewed pot with a tablespoon of fenugreek seeds and drink three times a day. If you are taking enough you will start to smell of maple syrup! Taking medicinal doses of fenugreek like this is not recommended during pregnancy or if you are taking anti-coagulant prescription medication. If you are diabetic, make sure that your insulin levels are well regulated before taking fenugreek.

Nettle tea is another easy herb to take to increase your milk, as are alfalfa sprouts. There is a full list on www.kellymom.com.

Don't use dummies while you get your breastfeeding established. Once your baby can find her hands easily, you can train her to suck her thumb.

Don't use cabbage leaves when you're trying to increase your milk supply (see page 133).

A major traumatic event in your life can interfere with the 'let-down' reflex. In the event of a serious shock or bereavement, keep your baby in close contact and let her suckle frequently to keep your milk flowing.

Bathing with your baby and taking her to bed with you will increase your milk supply. Skin-to-skin contact makes breastfeeding feel nicer and work better.

Enough for two? Or three?

How do you breastfeed twins? Fortunately, you are equipped with two nipples. Unfortunately, you only have one pair of hands.

The more your babies breastfeed, the more milk you will produce, so there's no physiological reason why a mother can't fully breastfeed twins, triplets or more. The first thing you'll need is confidence. Check the 'tricky babies' and the 'tricky nipples' sections on pages 50 to 53 to identify any potential areas of concern. Then get on with it.

However, multiple babies are usually small or premature, which may affect their ability to feed well in the first few weeks. If this is an issue then the second thing you'll need is a hospital-grade electric pump so that you can express milk for them, and build up your supply. (You can rent them, you don't have to buy them).

And the third thing that would be really useful is an extra pair of hands. Initially you'll want a helper to hold one baby in position on the breast, so you can get the second baby latched on well. Without this extra help, you may end up with inefficient feeding and sore nipples.

So if you haven't got a reliable supporter to help you, then get the fourth thing. Bottles, teats, lids and a steam steriliser. Feeding some bottles of expressed milk or (shock horror!) formula may help you to be in two places at once.

Unless you have help, you'll probably have to feed your babies one at a time at first. This takes longer, but it means that you can give each one the attention they need to learn to feed well. It's also a good time to concentrate on each baby's individual personality. To the rest of the world they may be 'the twins' or 'the triplets' or 'the quads', but to you, their mother, each baby is his own person, loved for his own self.

A practical consideration. Do you feed one baby from your first breast, then switch to the second breast after burping? Then attach the second baby to the second breast first, and then switch him to the first one? You need to swop the babies over so they don't grow lopsided. The babies, that is, not the breasts! Are you even going to remember which baby fed last, let alone which breast he fed from? It would help if they didn't look so similar.

Once your babies are latching on better, you can progress to feeding them two at a time. This is likely to be faster than single feeds, as the milk will let down strongly. If anyone out there is scoffing at the idea that a woman can breastfeed triplets, I'd like to point out that breastfeeding two babies while you bottle-feed the third is actually a better practical option than bottle-feeding three babies at once.

Life with multiple babies is one long continual round of feeding, expressing, burping, changing and comforting. Actually, life with any baby is one endless round of babycare, and at least with twins or triplets you *expect* to devote your entire life to the task. Still, you will want to do absolutely anything you can to make your life easier. So here are various 'rules' about breastfeeding single babies, together with my permission for you to ignore them in your special case.

Dummies are not recommended for a young breastfed baby, because they encourage carers to ignore early signs of hunger and artificially extend the time between feeds. Here you are with more than one baby. You're not ignoring the hungry one(s), but you can't actually feed him/them at the moment, because baby number one hasn't finished feeding yet. Sticking a dummy in a hungry baby's mouth could help him to stay happy for five minutes longer. You can always discontinue them if they affect his feeding.

Bottle-feeding is not recommended for young babies in case they get nipple confusion and refuse the breast. Admittedly, that's a risk, but if you're alone with two or more babies who don't yet feed well, then you can weigh that theoretical risk against the practical reality that one baby might be screaming for a feed for half an hour until you finish feeding his brother. So if you need to, you can forget about nipple confusion, express milk while you breastfeed and feed by bottle too in the early days. Breastfeeding will become easier in time, so you can phase this out. If one baby starts to favour the bottle over the breast, spend 24 hours breastfeeding that one with lots of skin contact and give the bottles to the other.

There are genuine reason why young babies shouldn't be fed *formula milk*: the gut flora of a purely breastfed baby is better if you don't feed any formula at all, and cow's milk is a common allergen. Your milk is best for your babies, and there is enough for your babies. However, if you feel that giving formula is going to make your life easier, then you can do that too. Start with one bottle a day. Your breasts get plenty of stimulation when you feed multiples, so this isn't likely to make your milk supply fail. (Remember that just because formula takes longer to digest than breastmilk, it isn't actually more satisfying for your baby.)

Formula supplements might be helpful or they might not. It can take time and effort to sterilise bottles and make up formula for your babies, only to find that your enthusiastic milk supply means that you have to express away the breastmilk they didn't drink.

Growth spurts are going to be particularly full-on when you're feeding more than one baby. Try to meet increased hunger with more breastfeeding, rather than more bottles of formula. Eat lots. Drink lots. Get lots of help.

You're meant to feed young babies whenever they're hungry, and let them sleep as long as they want to. Unless you have more than one. Getting simultaneous feeding established often means waking a sleeping baby to feed when his brother is hungry. Your babies won't necessarily have the same patterns of sleeping or feeding, so you may have to juggle their demands with your need to feed them both at once. Feeding on something approaching a three-hour schedule is the usual way to manage triplets.

In an ideal world, your babies would be able to finish all their breastfeeds in their own time. And you would be able to employ a full-time chef and housemaid for the daily chores. Still, try to keep sight of the idea that it's good for your babies to feed until they're full at some point in the day.

Skin-to-skin contact is important for multiples, just as it is for singletons. Bathing with your babies is also lovely, but you'll need another dry pair of hands to make it work.

Although breastfeeding your babies does make exclusive demands on your time and energy levels, everyone benefits in the long run. You'll be able to feed your babies instant, pre-warmed, perfect food, and you'll have cleverer, healthier, happy babies who you can comfort at the breast. It won't make mothering multiples easy, but it might make it easier.

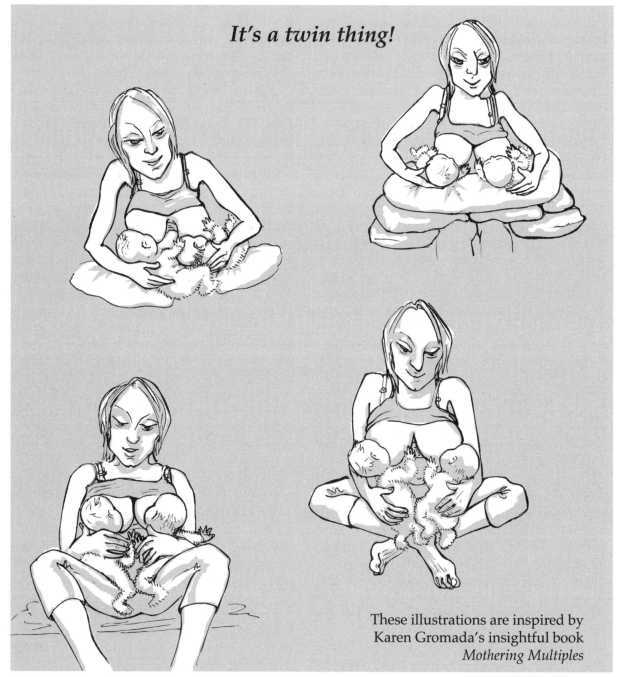

It's a twin thing!

These illustrations are inspired by Karen Gromada's insightful book *Mothering Multiples*

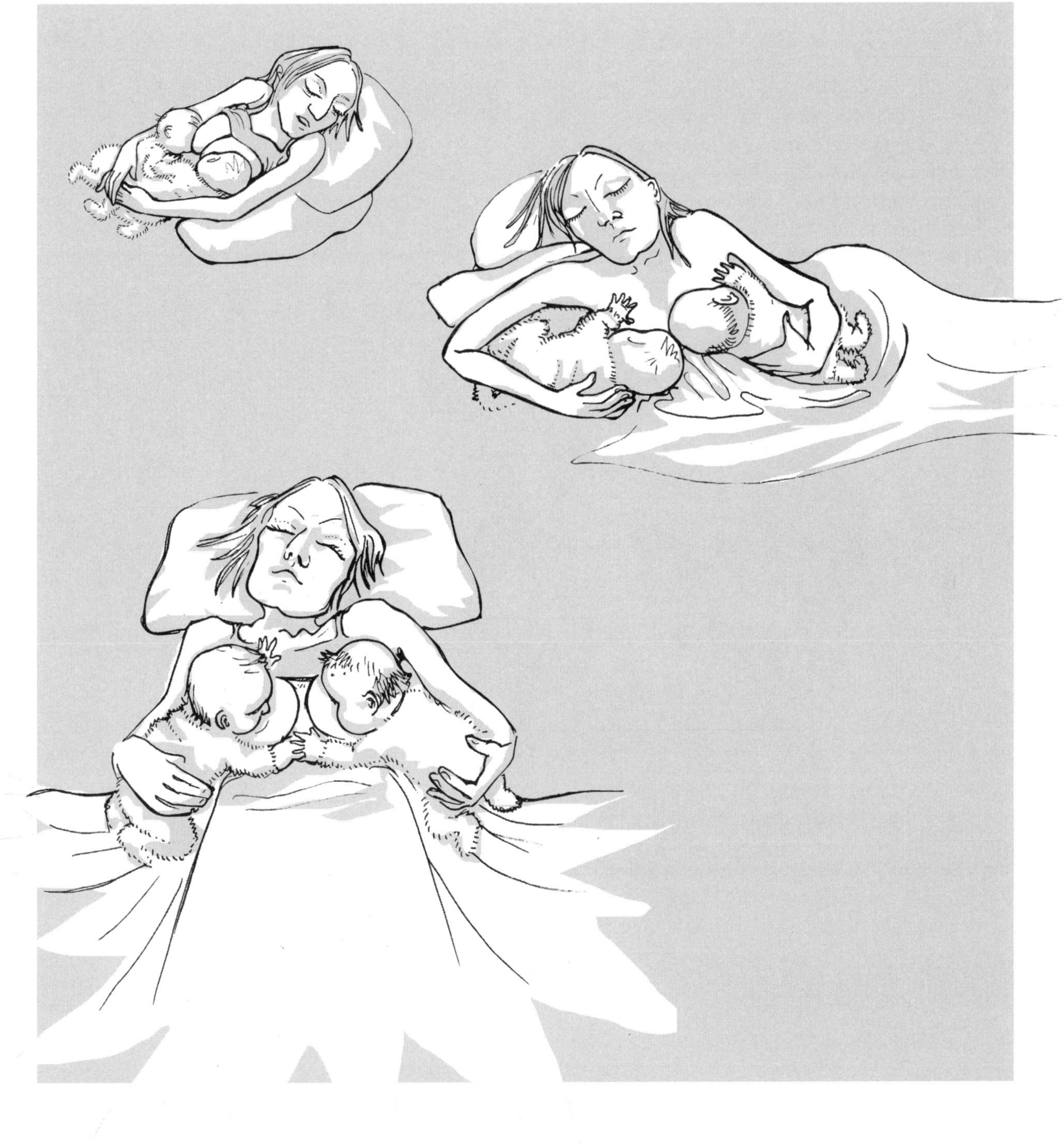

Oops, I appear to have too much milk!

For the first few days, your breasts produce little drops of creamy or clear colostrum.

You may find that when your milk comes in, on around the fourth day after the birth, that there's a lot of it. To be exact, it may feel like you've woken up with someone sitting on your chest.

This is a good survival strategy for the human race, but it's painful for you. Your body has geared up to produce vastly more milk than your baby needs, and will take a couple of days to calm down.

If your breasts are round, rock-hard all over and painful, then you are experiencing engorgement. This will correct itself over time – it's only by being full that your breasts get the message to reduce supply. Stick some cabbage leaves down your bra. Seriously! That is the recommended medical procedure in this situation! For more information on engorgement see page 133.

Some women experience milk flow that is so fast and efficient that a little baby will choke and splutter and come off the breast. If this happens repeatedly, then you can try leaning back during the feed. Sit up straight to attach the baby as usual, then carefully lean back, until the milk slows. You may need to end up lying on your back. Pay close attention to how the baby is latched on, so he doesn't drag your nipple sideways and cause the skin to crack.

If after a few weeks of breastfeeding you still have a ridiculously abundant milk supply, you can try block feeding[1]. Only do this if your breasts are continually becoming engorged, if the baby is refusing the breast, or if he has greenish, frothy poo (a sign that he is getting too much fore-milk and not enough rich hind-milk). First, use a mechanical breast pump to drain both breasts, then feed the baby off your 'empty' breasts – the hind-milk there will satisfy him. Now adopt a strategy of feeding from one breast as often as he wants for the next three hours. Switch to the other breast after this time. Carefully monitor the unused breast for blocked ducts (see page 139).

If three-hourly feeding blocks don't help the situation, you can repeat the pumping and increase the amount of time the baby feeds from one side to four, six, eight or even 12 hours at a time. This should solve the oversupply problem.

Some women who have too much milk express off the surplus and donate it to a milk bank. In the old days you would have been set up for life with a lucrative wet-nursing job.

Leaking milk is a common and embarrassing feature of feeding a tiny baby. One breast may drip milk while you are feeding from the other, milk may squirt everywhere after your baby has finished a feed, and most annoyingly, you can suddenly find that milk floods down the front of your shirt while you are miles away from your baby, thinking about something else entirely. Spookily, this sudden milk let down often happens at the exact moment that your baby wakes for a feed. And at lots of other times as well.

You can buy breast pads to put in your bra to soak up leakage. Disposable and washable sorts are both available. It can also help to press the heel of your hand firmly against a leaking nipple, to staunch the flow. Get a waterproof undersheet and sleep on some towels. Patterned clothes show up milk leakage less than plain clothes. Dark colours are better than light.

Don't worry, this stage will pass.

If you don't experience leaking milk or engorgement then that's fine. Lucky you. You still have enough milk. Honest.

How often should you feed yourself?

Making milk all day can be a strangely draining experience. It's a good idea to keep yourself topped up with savoury snacks during the day, to give yourself extra energy. Listen to your body, and try to include nutritious foods in your diet. Drink a little extra water if your pee goes dark.

You might be dismayed by the extra shapely figure that you have gained along with the baby, but now is not the time to go on a crash diet. Starving yourself can cause your milk supply to dwindle. You are giving extra calories to your baby every day, so give yourself time to let your figure adjust naturally. Some women seem to drop all the baby weight quite quickly while breastfeeding. But then some women seem to stay supersized the whole time, regardless of what they eat. If you think about it from your body's point of view, carrying a bit of extra weight is a good insurance policy against famine, so it might confer an evolutionary advantage to breastfeeding mothers. Damn.

Never mind. Next year you'll be rushing around trying to catch a toddler. The weight should drop off then.

If you want to lose weight, then do some regular exercise. You could also cut out sugary, processed food from your diet and switch to eating whole grains, pulses, vegetables, potatoes and protein-rich foods like meat, fish, tofu and nuts. *Don't cut out complex carbs*. The Atkins diet is incompatible with breastfeeding. The Low GI diet is more sensible. Read more about post-pregnancy body image on page 167.

There are plenty of magazines out there, going on and on (and on) about how the latest celebrity mum has got back to size zero within a month of the birth. Those poor women. They're not even allowed to be woman-shaped for just one year of special time with their baby. Instead they have to spend all hours in the gym in pursuit of plastic perfection. The answer to this is not to diet, it's to stop reading lifestyle magazines.

I eat a terrible diet – does that mean I shouldn't breastfeed?

No. Even poorly nourished women produce nutritious breastmilk. Researchers in the Gambia studied women who were eating a poor subsistence diet and measured the nutritional content of their milk. Then they gave them supplements. The quality of their milk didn't change[1]. Your milk will still be good enough if you don't eat well; however, you will be healthier and have more energy if you do.

It's easier to eat healthily if you do it positively rather than negatively. Get some healthy food and include it in your diet. Don't sit around stressing about how you really want a chocolate biscuit, and it would be REALLY BAD to eat it. That's only going to make you want it more.

My list of favourite, easy-to-eat, good foods includes smoothies, steamed veg drizzled with olive oil, mackerel, hummus, watercress and tahini. I also recommend Floradix iron supplement and spirulina powder dissolved in pineapple juice (tasty, but very green). That might turn you on, or alternatively you might now decide that I'm the Anti-Christ. Make your own list of good foods, and give yourself good points for eating them.

Alcohol interferes with the natural high you get from breastfeeding. Normally, when you breastfeed it's the feel-good hormone oxytocin that gets your milk flowing. After just one drink, oxytocin levels drop, your breasts become less efficient, and your milk production over the next two hours decreases by 23%[2].

Drinking alcohol will not make your baby sleep better. Clinical trials have shown that after one drink, the babies of lactating mothers sleep more fitfully and wake more[3].

The alcohol that passes into your milk isn't enough to make your baby drunk, but it doesn't have to be much to do some damage. One study has shown that the babies of mothers who drink every day, or who drink to get drunk, have delayed motor development at one year[4].

Having said that, drinking alcohol while breastfeeding isn't as harmful as drinking while pregnant. Women who abuse alcohol in their pregnancy can give their babies brain damage. You probably found that your body got the message when you were pregnant, and just the thought of a can of beer made you want to be sick. Now the baby's out, though, it's all changed, and it's quite possible that you could really fancy a drink.

You can still have a drink. You can have two units of alcohol after a feed. That's a large glass of wine, a can of beer, or a double measure of spirits. The alcohol will have completely cleared from your milk in three hours[5]. (Expressing and discarding your milk won't make this happen any quicker[6].) You can still feed your baby in the meantime, and as long as you don't do this every day then your baby won't be harmed. But don't drink enough to get drunk.

You may find this easy, or it might take a lot of willpower. Heavy drinking is horrendously common in British society. You might really miss the social crutch of alcohol.

Mind you, once you spend some time reflecting on what an idiot you used to make of yourself when you were drunk, you may find you don't miss it so much after all.

Make a small amount of alcohol go a very long way by mixing soda water with your wine, for a weak spritzer, or making shandy out of your beer. That way you don't have to feel left out. It may help to make yourself a special soft drink. You can spend some money on a nice smoothie or a lush hot chocolate, or you can mix fruit juice with fizzy water for a refreshingly cheap special drink.

There is another reason why you may want to swear off alcohol completely. There is some evidence that alcoholism is inherited[7]. The taste of anything you eat or drink travels into your breastmilk[8] and teaches your baby that that is a safe, desirable flavour. If your parents or your partner has a drinking problem then think about whether you want your baby to learn to like whisky or beer at your breast.

You also can't drink at all if you or your baby has thrush. See pages 136–137.

The problem with giving women the advice that a SMALL amount of alcohol is okay, is that people twist your words. One glass of wine is not a bottle. Half a pint of beer is not half a pint of vodka. If you know that once you start drinking, then you can't stop, then just *don't go there*.

If you really want to go out and get drunk, then express some milk ahead of time and leave your baby with an all-night baby sitter. You may well find your breasts fill up while you're out and you need to hand-express milk onto some paper in the toilets. Still, you'll look great in a low-cut top. You've just had a year off alcohol, so you are now Officially a Lightweight. *Do not drink as much as your friends*. Drink plenty of extra soft drinks and water. Making milk dehydrates you, and dehydration can turn a small amount of alcohol into a terrible hangover.

And you can learn to have a good time without drinking. You can't take your baby to a pub in the evening, but you can go to the cinema together, or out for a meal, or round to visit a friend. Lots of yummy breastfeeds and snuggles will keep your baby quiet. Good company and good times can be had without propping up the bar.

The active ingredient in **Cannabis**, THC, is fat-soluble, so it is stored in fatty tissue, including in your breasts. It does pass into your milk[9] and frequent use can depress your milk supply. The children of heavy cannabis smokers have smaller heads than other children[10]. As with alcohol, there is some evidence that children of cannabis smokers have delayed motor development at one year. Like with alcohol, if you smoke cannabis there is some risk to your baby, although your milk will still be better for your child than formula.

Don't take ecstasy, cocaine, ketamine, heroin or speed or abuse tranquillisers while breastfeeding. These are all highly toxic substances which could kill your baby or make her very ill. Stay off the hallucinogens. Life is one big trip for a tiny baby; she doesn't need it to be enhanced.

Cigarettes are really bad (and if you're a smoker then reading that sentence probably made you want to smoke one!). Cigarette smoke contains known toxins such as carbon monoxide and lead. While alcohol or cannabis in your breastmilk could stunt your baby's development, smoking near your baby could kill him. Babies whose mothers smoke run twice the risk of dying of cot death.[11] Never, ever smoke around your baby, or in the room where your baby sleeps.

By smoking, you are also increasing the risk of your child contracting asthma, bronchitis, pneumonia and ear infections leading to partial deafness. Your child is also more likely to be burnt in a fire.[12]

Hey, presumably you've heard this before. If you've still smoked all the way through pregnancy, despite all the pleadings and threats of the medical establishment, then you're pretty heavily addicted. Still, now might be another good time to give up. Hypnotherapy can help you to stop. It's expensive, but then so is smoking. Or find more support and ideas online. Nicotine patches are safe to use while breastfeeding.[13]

But, if you have tried and failed, and you can't stop smoking yet, then congratulate yourself for breastfeeding. Breastfed babies in smoking households go on to have fewer illnesses than children who were bottle-fed.[14]

Caffeine is a drug. Some babies are fine when their mothers drink caffeine, but it can keep a baby awake, and might make him irritable. It's crazy really: your baby is awake all night, so you have to drink loads of coffee to make it through the day, and then the baby is awake all night again.[15]

Many women don't really want to drink coffee when they're pregnant. Like with alcohol, though, you pretty quickly feel the urge to get back into your old bad habits once the baby is born. Maybe keep your coffee consumption low for a couple of months, until you know what normal sleeping is for your baby? Tea is lower in caffeine, so shouldn't be too problematic.

If you currently can't function without coffee, but think it might not be helping your baby, you can try substituting an increasing amount of decaf into the mix, slowly, over a period of weeks. Tea, cola, Iron Bru and Lucozade also contain caffeine, as do some extra strength painkillers. Avoid Red Bull.

Some *prescription drugs* are unsafe to take while breastfeeding. Don't expect your doctor to remember this. Always remind her that you are breastfeeding when she prescribes medication for you. You can double-check with the pharmacist when you pick up the prescription.

Don't worry...

That was a lot of 'don'ts'. Well, hey, the rest of the population don't get doses of natural oxytocin and prolactin all day and night. These feel-good chemicals come free with breastfeeding. If you could get them on prescription, everyone would want them.

Having a baby isn't going to be the last time you have fun.

You don't have to worry about eating spicy or strongly flavoured foods when you breastfeed. Yes, the flavour comes through in the milk, but babies like that.

You don't have to worry about pollutants in the environment coming through in your breastmilk. Cows are fed agricultural chemicals every day, so formula milk is far worse.

You don't have to drink milk to make milk. You can if you want to, but you don't have to. No other mammals do.

Unless...

Now this isn't very common, but it is possible for your baby to be allergic to food substances that pass into your breastmilk. Consider this if your baby is feeding well, yet consistently fails to gain weight, if she has eczema or asthma, a permanently runny nose or ear infections, colicky digestive pain[16], lots of wind, or persistent red nappy rash around the anus or diarrhoea.

Giving up breastfeeding is likely to make everything worse, as cows' milk is a common allergen. If your child is having some bottles of formula, then try to phase these out or switch to a hypoallergenic formula.

Next, try an exclusion diet. This is best conducted with the support of your doctor or a recommended nutritionist. Foods that people commonly develop reactions to include wheat, milk and milk products, yeast, nuts, eggs, shellfish, food additives, chocolate, tomatoes and citrus fruit. First, try excluding any foods that you're suspicious about. If that doesn't work, move to a strict diet of a few safe foods. (If your doctor can't suggest one, consult an allergy specialist or book on the subject.) My, this will be dull. Reintroduce other foods slowly over a period of weeks.

Don't try doing this over Christmas, as it would probably give you a nervous breakdown.

I know exclusion diets are difficult. I've done this myself. But it's really worth trying to pinpoint food sensitivities at an early age. If your child is highly allergic to a major food in her diet, then eating it throughout her childhood could stunt her growth. On the other hand, if you spot the problem food early, and keep her off it for a few years, she might grow out of the allergy in later life.

How often should you feed your baby?

'By two weeks, your baby… should manage to last three to four hours between feeds.'
The New Contented Little Baby Book
by Gina Ford

'THE INFANT SHOULD BE PUT TO THE BREAST AT REGULAR INTERVALS OF ABOUT FOUR HOURS'
CHAMBERS' ENCYCLOPEDIA
VOL 10, 1880

'A baby that is latched on correctly will rarely need to spend more than an hour feeding.'
What to Expect When You're Breastfeeding — And What if You Can't?
by Clare Byam-Cook

'If he were suckled at stated periods he would only look for it at those times, and be satisfied.'
Advice to Wife and Mother,
by Pye Henry Chavasse MD
1872

Your baby is very unlikely to have read any of these books.

Feed your baby when he's hungry, and feed him until he's had enough.

Some people call that 'feeding on demand'. What a daft phrase. He's not being demanding. He's not trying to 'manipulate' you, or to 'get you to react'. He's tiny, he's vulnerable and he has a stomach the size of a golf ball. He's hungry. Feed him.

What if he just wants comfort? So, comfort him! If he wants the breast, that's fine. If your baby isn't allowed some comfort in the first few months of his life, then when is he ever going to get some?

Feeding hunger is the best way to establish successful breastfeeding. Your breasts work on a supply and demand basis. However much the baby suckles at one feed, that's how much they 'expect' to make the next time round. Your breasts have to keep up with the needs of a growing infant. You are the sole life support system for a tiny, voracious person who is going to double his weight in a matter of months. That's why when he's hungry, you feed him.

I found this one pretty simple. My baby

settled into a pattern of wake up, feed, play, feed, sleep. I spent an incredible amount of time breastfeeding, which was fine, because I'm basically quite lazy. The baby got fat.

Breastfeeding is a natural way for a baby to go to sleep. After all, your milk has delta-sleep-inducing-peptide in it. Sure, feeding my baby to sleep meant that he expected to go to sleep feeding a lot. That didn't really bother me. I figured I was his mum, and I wasn't going anywhere.

It's not that straightforward with all babies. Some babies get crabby, the mother wonders what on earth she's doing wrong, and may well feel subtly blamed by hippy earth mothers like me who float around saying 'Oh, it's easy – you just feed the baby lots'.

Sometimes there is a medical cause for excessive crying, so get your baby seen by a doctor. An internet search for 'colic' or 'reflux' may help make sense of your baby's symptoms. If she is suffering from colic, then cutting out dairy products from your diet may help (see page 81). Reflux is helped by frequent breastfeeds, and by being carried upright in a sling. Difficult babies, particularly if they have been through a difficult birth, often benefit from seeing a craniosacral therapist or chiropractor.

Cranky babies are often overstimulated and overtired, and might benefit from quiet times where you have to help them to sleep. Tracy Hogg (who I disagree with on some issues) advises in her book *The Baby Whisperer* that you institute a pattern of wake up, feed, play, sleep. It works for some babies, who will fall asleep calmly once you recognise their tired signs (yawning, turning away from toys) as long as you intervene before they become overtired.

But hang on, Tracy Hogg is a nursery nurse: she's very good at getting babies to sleep without breastfeeding, because that's her job. Sure, some babies don't need to be breastfed to sleep, and you can experiment with different sleep strategies to find the one that works for your child. But if your baby is crying and you know that the breast will calm him, bear in mind that maybe he's right, and the books are wrong.

Give yourself time and space to learn your baby. If he's crying, he's either hungry, or tired, or overtired, or freaked out, or in pain, or has wind. He'll have different cries for different scenarios, except for hunger and wind which, confusingly, can sound exactly the same. An older baby will add an 'I'm bored, play with me' cry to his repertoire. Newborn babies don't do this.

Basically, the baby indicates 'jump' and you respond with 'how high?'. That's a psychologically healthy and appropriate relationship between a small baby and his carer. Exactly what you need to do when he says 'jump' is a voyage of discovery, although in my experience, it generally involved unhooking my bra.

Breastmilk helps with more than just hunger. It eases pain, dilutes reflux, quenches thirst, fights infections, aids sleep and calms jangled nerves. If it's not working for your baby, then try something else, but if it is then don't knock it.

Part of your job involves responding to your baby's needs, the other part involves anticipating his needs. It can take weeks for you to both start to click in together. Sometimes he will be freaked out because you will be freaked out because it's all too much. There will always be days when things don't go right between you, although they'll hopefully be balanced by days where they do. There is no such thing as a perfect mother.

Chuck out the clock

You're doing a vital job when you spend all day just hanging out with your baby. Psychologist Naomi Stadlen has written a brilliant book *What Mothers Do*, in which she lists all the things that mothers do with their babies that we don't even have words for. So many mothers think that they haven't got anything done with their day, when they have, they've put their time in to make a whole new happy person.

I can't tell you how often to feed your baby because I don't know how hungry your baby will be. But I do know that sitting there watching the clock is going to make breastfeeding a more frustrating experience. Babies don't do very much when they feed. They pause, they flutter, they pause a while more. You can't really hurry them up – you have to slow down to match. If you want to, you can note what time of day your baby likes to feed. If you are an organised person who likes some structure to the day then you can draw up all kinds of charts and tables showing when your baby likes to do what. Or you can drift along, taking each day as it comes. Either approach is fine.

What isn't OK is making a hungry baby wait to feed until some book says that a suitable time has elapsed. Remember, *your baby hasn't read those books*. Did you think that your baby was only going to be hungry every four hours? I wonder where that idea came from?

There has been a lot of absolute rubbish written about childcare over the last 200 years, most of it by men, and very little of it by mothers.

The nineteenth and twentieth centuries saw great advances in medical science; amazing leaps in our understanding of such things as germs, disease transmission, anaesthesia and surgery. Unfortunately, this was accompanied by the medicalisation of babycare, which removed and distanced women from their babies.

The idea, the doctors thought, was simple. A baby is a blank slate, in effect a little machine. If you programme it to feed every four hours, it will. If you 'give in' and allow it to 'dictate' its unreasonable demands, then you have made a rod for your own back, and you'll be running after it day and night. Be firm, and teach that baby to be more reasonable. Stop that mollycoddling, and instill it with independence from an early age. This school of thought is still prevalent in popular attitudes to childcare today, and it's based on a fundamental misunderstanding of human psychology.

A baby's needs are entirely unreasonable. He has no sense of time. He doesn't know that in another twenty minutes, his food will be coming. All he has is HUNGRY and NOW. If you don't pick up on his hungry face, and little hungry noises, then he has to do hungry CRYING, and that's all he can do to get food.

The doctors noted that when they prevented the mother from answering those cries, the baby eventually stopped bothering to make them. So their theory worked. When a mother only suckled an infant at stated periods he did learn not to cry when he was hungry. And he learned a very harsh lesson about life for one so young – that you can't expect your basic needs to be met. Maybe the child somehow managed to be satisfied even when he was hungry. Or maybe, he was just deeply depressed.

You can't teach your baby to be reasonable.

Reason is something he will learn much later, well after he has grasped such concepts as cause and effect.

You also can't teach your baby to be independent. Your child, as he grows older, will naturally become independent, all on his own, as he branches out and does new things, because he is happy and contented and secure in your love. You can't force independence, he has to choose it.

Here's an analogy. If you want to, you can choose solitude. You can sit in your bedroom and meditate for a week. However, if someone were to *force* solitude upon you by installing a lock on the outside of your bedroom door, then that would no longer be solitude – it would be imprisonment.

It's just the same with child development; forced independence isn't real independence, it's abandonment. And when you're tiny and helpless, and your parents are your only means of surviving in this world, abandonment is very scary indeed.

At the same time as strict, four-hourly feeding schedules started to be advocated, bottle-feeding became more popular. I wonder why? So it takes twenty minutes for a baby to digest breastmilk, but how long does it take for her to digest formula milk again? Oh yes, that's right. Four hours. What a *good* baby, not crying between meals.

Four hours is the maximum that a newborn baby should go without a feed, measured from the beginning of one feed to the next. And when a breastfeeding mother makes herself wait between feeds, her breasts get full, they get the message that they're overproducing, so they scale down milk production. Although women and babies have survived breastfeeding regimes which space and limit feeds, optimum breastfeeding occurs when she stays in closer contact with her baby's dietary requirements.

One modern version of the old-school strict baby routine addresses the problem of diminishing supply by getting mothers to express milk as well as breastfeeding.

Routine for a breast-feeding baby at one week:
7am
– Baby should be awake, nappy changed and feeding no later than 7am.
– He needs 25-35 minutes on the full breast, then offer 10-15 minutes on the second breast after you have expressed 60-90ml.
– Do not feed after 8am, as it will put baby off his next feed.

The New Contented Little Baby Book

You could do this. If you wanted to, you could rise at the crack of dawn and sterilise a bottle, assemble a breast pump while your child is crying, try to calm him on schedule, feed him a little (but not necessarily enough to get much satisfying hind-milk) and then put him down to scream while you attempt to express milk from your breast. Or you could stay in bed and feed your baby.

Books that tell you when to do what to your baby are very popular. Partly this is because many women in modern society have no experience whatsoever of babies, before suddenly being handed their own. It is reassuring to find that you can buy an instruction manual that tells you something more specific than just 'go with whatever your baby says he needs' (basically, my position).

But really, it's because women today are doing an impossible job...

Human beings are a tribal species. Just as surely as fish swim in shoals and wildebeest run in herds, we have evolved to live in a close-knit, extended family group. There is a common saying in many countries that 'it takes a village to raise a child', and if we were living as we used to live, at least twenty other people would be actively helping you and your partner to look after this baby.

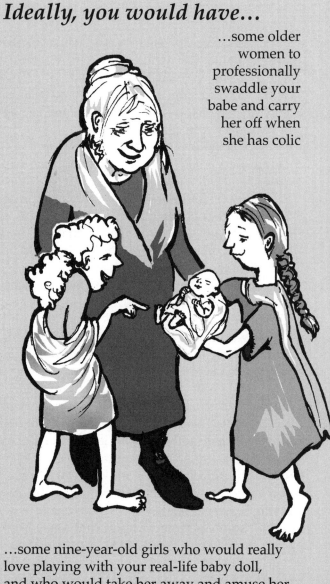

Ideally, you would have...

...some older women to professionally swaddle your babe and carry her off when she has colic

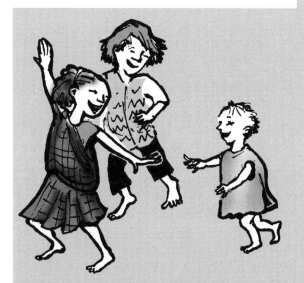

...a gang of children excitedly playing together. As soon as your toddler could walk, she would run off and join them

...some nine-year-old girls who would really love playing with your real-life baby doll, and who would take her away and amuse her for long periods. Children love babies, and babies love children

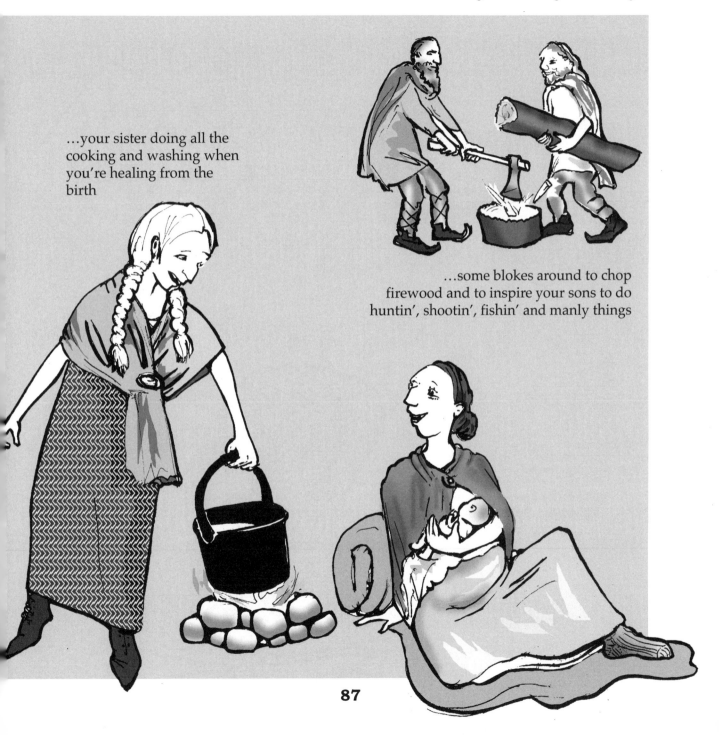

...your sister doing all the cooking and washing when you're healing from the birth

...some blokes around to chop firewood and to inspire your sons to do huntin', shootin', fishin' and manly things

87

Instead, you have...

...pizza delivery, for
your emergency
dinner needs

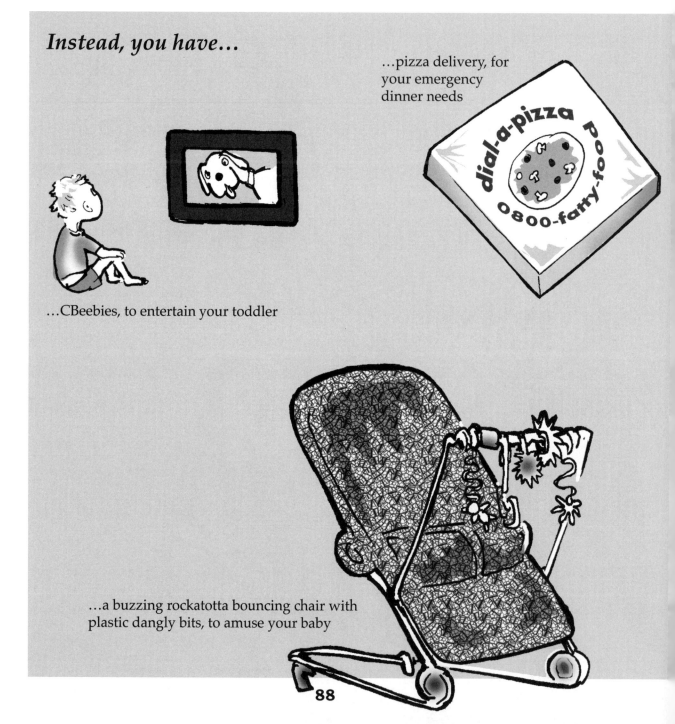

...CBeebies, to entertain your toddler

...a buzzing rockatotta bouncing chair with
plastic dangly bits, to amuse your baby

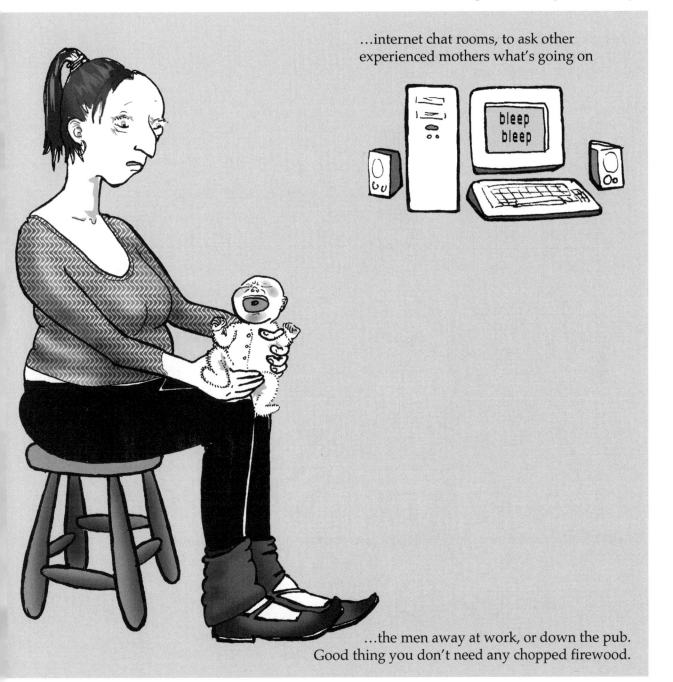

...internet chat rooms, to ask other experienced mothers what's going on

...the men away at work, or down the pub. Good thing you don't need any chopped firewood.

The problem with our modern way of life is that babies prefer human company to plastic, bouncing, rockatotta baby seats.

This is why:

Human evolution: scenario 1

Once upon a time, a baby was born who was quite happy to be left alone for long periods of time. He sat gurgling beneath a banyan tree…

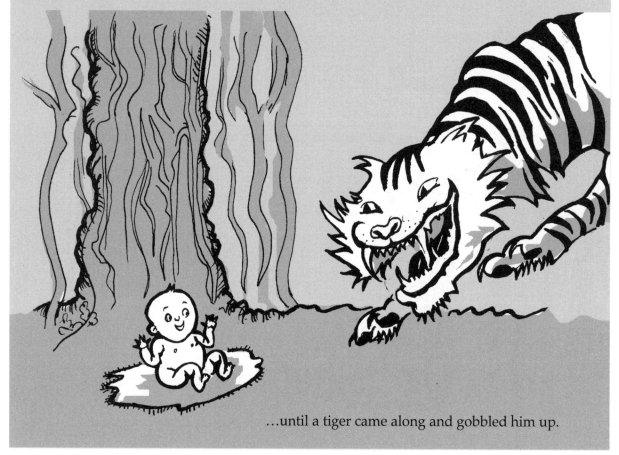

…until a tiger came along and gobbled him up.

Human evolution: scenario 2

Around the same time, another baby was born. Every time his mother tried to put him down, he screamed as if a tiger was about to attack him…

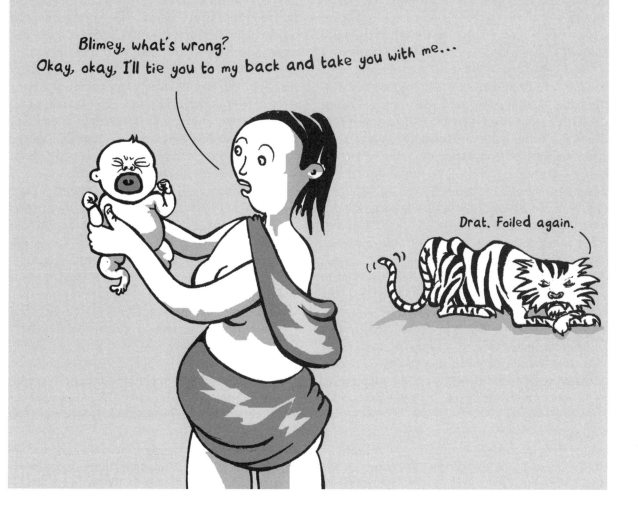

Guess which baby yours is descended from?

Human babies are extraordinarily needy. If our babies were as physiologically developed as say, a gazelle's baby, then you would be giving birth to a walking talking toddler who would be ready for preschool. But we are not gazelles. We walk upright, which means we have a smaller pelvic opening, and we have large brains, which make for bigger heads. So we have to give birth to our babies when they are still very tiny, and developmentally helpless.

For most of our evolutionary history, our babies have been carried by loving members of the tribe. Predators were a real risk. Constant carrying kept babies safe. It seems likely that the first clothes humans developed were baby slings, adopted to bind their babies to their hairless bodies.

Mothers weren't expected to care for their babies on their own. Human beings and whales are the only species to have a menopause. Every other kind of animal, including chimpanzees, remain fertile until the day they die. Those older, wiser, infertile grandmothers evolved to help us with our needy babies.[1]

So, your baby doesn't know that she's 'meant' to sleep alone in a cot. She doesn't know that she really should like the fancy bouncy chair that you spent so much money on. Human contact feels good to her, and she's going to want lots of it, because that is how babies have always survived.

Assuming that you're on your own with your baby for much of the day, your baby is likely to want you to hold her for much of the time. Unfortunately, unlike all the relatives and other village members who should be sharing this task, you smell lovely and milky. So, while you're holding her, she might opportunistically remind you that she'd like a little snack. Therefore, you are likely to do a lot of breastfeeding, possibly more often than the mother with the extended network of impromptu babysitters.

The way that our society is structured makes life difficult for mothers. Up until the late eighteenth century, family life, home life and work life in Britain were integrated. You worked alongside your children, and they grew up helping you with your tasks. This was still tribal living, with the flexibility for many different people to interact with, and be responsible for the baby over the course of the day. Then came industrialisation. Men went off to the offices and factories. Children were herded off to school. Women were left holding the baby.

Throughout the nineteenth century, most women worked from home, and juggled domestic drudgery, childcare and piecework or laundry to supplement their income. In the late twentieth century, we won the right to go out to work with men on equal terms, and with a stab at equal pay.

But this hasn't actually made life any easier for the mothers of young babies. Back in the drearily tedious world of the 1950s housewife, women could at least depend on there being other mothers around nearby. Most neighbourhoods consisted of networks of women actively supporting each other in their endeavours.

Nowadays, the vast majority of women work outside the home. This means that your identity and your social network is likely to be bound up with your job. Once you've left on maternity leave, you no longer see a whole swathe of people who are socially important for you.

You probably don't know your neighbours, or because they're out at work all day, they aren't around to help. You are likely to have moved away from your parents and sisters so you or your partner can find work. You're on your own. That's the problem.

So what do women do to try and manage the impossible job of meeting their own and their babies' needs alone?

Strict babycare routines have been developed by nursery nurses and other childcare professionals to try and reduce a baby's dependence on his carers. If you do exactly the same thing at exactly the same time each day, then the baby does expect sleeping and eating to only happen at these intervals. This theoretically gives the mother more time off, but it also ties her into a very rigid pattern for her days.

The guesswork is taken out of parenting. You no longer have to respond to your baby's cues, instead you simply anticipate everything your baby might need, before he has a chance to ask for it. These routines are designed to be implemented from the first week of a baby's life. You could train a puppy to live in a box if you did it from the first week of its life. That doesn't make it natural.

If you do opt for a very structured parenting routine, and you want your breastfeeding to succeed (and, let's face it, breastfeeding isn't the be all and end all of motherhood, it's just a healthy, lovely bit) then delay imposing feeding schedules until you have been feeding well for three months.

But there are other ways of raising a baby. It cuts me up that there are mothers out there who feel they are failing, or that their baby is 'difficult' because he doesn't feed or sleep at the times some book says he should. We're all different, babies included.

Because babycare routines are so popular, they dominate people's ideas of how you are meant to bring up a baby. 'What's your routine?' my sister was asked.

'Er, my mum comes round on a Thursday.'

Plenty of babies survive just fine with very little in the way of a structured routine. Some need nap times, others just fall asleep on the breast. If you have one of those babies who is happy to be hoicked around with you in a sling all day, then you can start to discover some of the advantages of *not* following a routine with your baby.

I drove a camper van across Spain with my son when he was six months old, and we had a brilliant time. Routine? What routine? When do I next feed my baby? At the next lay-by! My baby slept happily through Spanish fiestas.

I could never count on my son going down in his cot for a set amount of time, while I got on with other things. Instead, he was usually in close contact with me or his dad. It was like there was still an umbilical cord there connecting us. And I really liked it like that. I breastfed him and we carried him and slept with him a lot. It was straightforward, and worked very well for me.

When I wanted a break, I recreated those old tribal networks and found a friend to take him for a bit. Many men, in particular, have never had a chance to hold a baby. They won't volunteer to take yours out of an understandable fear that its wobbly, squashy head might fall off. However, if you plonk the baby on them and explain the basic way to hold it, they can have some lovely baby time, and you can have some lovely not-baby time.

Spontaneous parenting depends on you being more available for your baby than structured parenting, but it brings its own rewards. When you're breastfeeding easily, and carrying your baby around with you, and if you don't bother faffing around with breastpumps and bottles and blackout blinds and cots, then you're a very portable package. So you and your baby can go out and have more fun.

However much structure you and your baby need, the key thing is to be responsive to your baby.

The good news is that, contrary to popular belief, responsive parenting actually makes your job easier. The childcare 'experts' told women that if they rushed to pick up their babies, they would learn to cry more. That's the exact opposite of what actually, initially happens.

If a mother consistently fails to pick up on a baby's subtle, non-verbal cues, and waits until her baby has been crying for some time before she attends to him, then the baby learns to cry more, and louder, any time he has a need that must be met. Feeling hungry? Don't waste time hanging around frowning and eating the blanket, no, SCREAM – NOW AND FOR AGES – that's how you get fed. If turning away from that unpleasantly bright sunshine doesn't work then accompany it with a very loud SCREAM. Straight away.

You can see this in a study[2] that compared mothers of young babies in London and in Copenhagen in 2006. The British mothers tended to respond slowly to their babies. They delayed going to their crying child about forty per cent of the time and the distressed babies were left without contact for up to an hour a day. The Danish mothers promptly answered their babies' cries, and the total amount of time the babies were left to cry without being held was only about 15 minutes in every 24 hours.

By the time they were just ten days old, the British babies in the survey had learned to cry more. Fifty per cent more. That's a lot. And the British mothers still had to spend just as much time feeding and caring for their babies, so that crying was completely pointless. The effects lasted. Their babies still cried more at five weeks and at 12 weeks of age.

The study only followed the babies for 12 weeks. Presumably, some of these babies might have gone on to learn that there's no point in screaming, and stopped. But I hope not.

Responsive parenting is the key to having happy children. If you regard a child's needs as unreasonable demands that should be ignored, then that will mess them up emotionally in one of two ways.

Your child could learn to exaggerate their needs to get your attention. Here lies the paradox that people who try and train their children to be independent before they are ready end up with really whiny, clingy kids.

Alternatively your child could learn to swallow his needs, and never to express them. This results in a kind of emotional detachment, where he can never really be in touch with his feelings, because deep down, he knows that it is unacceptable to have any.

Does this sound extreme? It has been scientifically verified in laboratory tests.

Attachment theory [3]

Mary Ainsworth, a developmental psychologist, spent a lot of time in the 1960s studying pairs of mothers and babies in Africa and in the USA. What she was studying was the quality of the bond between the two, and she paid particular attention to how responsive a mother was to her baby's cues. From this, she developed the Strange Situation Test. An eleven-month-old baby was briefly left with a stranger in a laboratory, and then his reaction was studied when he was reunited with his mother.

The Strange Situation Test can be used to divide mother/baby pairs into three broad categories of bond or 'attachment'. Some of the babies were upset when their mother left the room, but when she came back, they accepted comfort from her and quietened down quickly. These babies had mothers who were prompt, consistent and appropriate in their attentions. They could trust their mothers to meet their needs. They played happily. They were 'securely attached'.

The other babies, the 'insecurely attached' ones, reacted in two different ways. Some babies were incredibly distressed when their mother left the room, and when she returned they were angry with her and slow to start playing again. They had mothers who were inconsistent. Sometimes she would answer their needs but at other times, for whatever reason, she would be unable to. So they lived in a state of permanent anxiety. Their negative emotions were exaggerated. They were 'ambivalently attached'.

And the third group were really worrying. These 'avoidantly attached' babies showed little or no emotion when their mother left them. There was no response when she came back either. That level of independence at such a young age is not good. These babies had learned that their mothers were not around to meet their emotional needs, so they just stopped displaying any. But those feelings were still in there, bubbling away. They couldn't explore and play as well as the other children. The effort of controlling their emotions didn't leave them much energy for learning.

Generations of social scientists have had the opportunity to study what happens next to insecurely attached infants. At preschool, the securely attached children turned out to be happy, fun, sociable, popular and intelligent. The anxiously attached kids acted babyish for their age – their extreme mood swings often interfered with their ability to learn. The avoidantly attached children bullied others at school – unable to access their own unhappy feelings, they felt no empathy for the hurt of others.

These children were not being abused. (There is a fourth category, 'disorganised attachment' for babies who are actually scared of their carers.) The mothers in all three groups were meeting their children's needs for food and shelter. Most of the mothers were affectionate, and few were overtly hostile. *All these mothers loved their children*. They all held their children for about the same amount of time overall. However, there was one big qualitative difference in what they did when they picked their babies up. The mothers of the insecurely attached babies never picked their babies up *when the babies signalled that they wanted to be held*.

More than a third of babies in the UK and in the US can be classed as insecurely attached.[4]

These babies grow up to be adults who have problems with work, with relationships, and with their mental health. As a society, we are failing to raise emotionally well-adjusted children. And still mothers here are isolated, unsupported, and encouraged to ignore their hungry babies for hours at a time.

You have nothing to lose, and everything to gain, by being as responsive to your baby as you can. Try to keep the attitude that he's allowed to cry and be demanding, and yes, it's difficult, but that's not your baby's fault. Take support where you can. Don't be afraid to ask for help. It's normal to think that because it's so hard, you must be doing something wrong. But babies are also amazing and wonderful, and they don't stay babies for long.

You can experiment with ways to make it easier for you too. You'll probably have to at some point – if not with your first child then certainly with your second.

Check that your attachment and positioning are good. A baby that is latched on well is feeding most efficiently. Sometimes you can feel the 'draw' as milk is drained from the breast at the beginning of a feed. Offer both breasts at each feed to let her fill herself up as much as she can in one go. Try breast compression (page 71) if you're irritated by her feeding slowly. If you still feel that your baby is feeding excessively, get your breastfeeding evaluated by a specialist. She will be able to offer you practical advice tailored to your situation.

Once your breastfeeding is established, it becomes more flexible. If you spend three months feeding your baby lots, then your milk won't dry up if you introduce the odd bottle of formula. (There's more about mixed feeding on page 180.) Try expressing milk so someone else can feed her if you want to experience the giddy feeling of lightness you get when you leave the house alone (see page 161). Both these strategies make breastfeeding easier for some mothers. Other women find exclusive breastfeeding easier, because they don't have to sterilise anything.

Your milk supply will work best if you feed your baby until she finishes her feed herself. However, this isn't always practically possible. Start off with this policy and find out for yourself how much breastfeeding your baby is capable of! Then once you are confident about the dynamics of breastfeeding and can see that she's gaining weight, you can experiment with cutting feeds short. One way to gauge this is to look at her little arms. She might start the feed with them all scrunched up, holding or sometimes pummelling the breast (which actually massages it and increases the milk flow – clever thing!). Then she'll settle down to the long business of obtaining nutrition. Her arms will gradually lose their tension, and start to drift away from your breast. Once they're down by her sides, you can assume she's almost done. Switch her to the other breast if she wants it – if not, hooray! put her down and creep away…

It's still a good idea to let her finish some feeds herself. Particularly if there's something good on telly.

How often should you feed your baby?

A lot.

You can't overfeed a breastfed baby. She can be as fat as a piglet and still be totally and utterly, completely healthy. It's true.

Things to do when you're breastfeeding – part 1

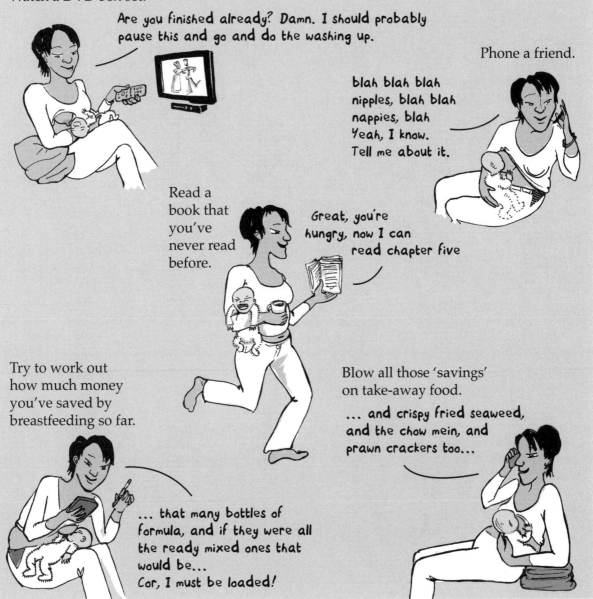

Watch a DVD box set.

Are you finished already? Damn. I should probably pause this and go and do the washing up.

Phone a friend.

blah blah blah nipples, blah blah nappies, blah Yeah, I know. Tell me about it.

Read a book that you've never read before.

Great, you're hungry, now I can read chapter five

Try to work out how much money you've saved by breastfeeding so far.

Blow all those 'savings' on take-away food.

... and crispy fried seaweed, and the chow mein, and prawn crackers too...

... that many bottles of formula, and if they were all the ready mixed ones that would be... Cor, I must be loaded!

97

Things to do when you're breastfeeding – part 2

Watch a DVD box set.

Yes, good idea. Let's watch 'The Blobbles go on Holiday' again. Anything for an easy life.

Phone a friend, while holding a simultaneous conversation with your toddler.

This is all part of a scientific experiment to discover how many different ways I can multitask without leaving the sofa

Read a book that you've read several hundred times before.

And the wolf huffed and he puffed and he puffed and he huffed and he yawned and he gazed out of the window and he cursed Hans Christian Andersen...

Try to work out how much money you've saved by breastfeeding so far.

let mummy do the calculator now... no, now...

Remember that you already spent that money on your oldest child's Christmas present.

Night feedzzz

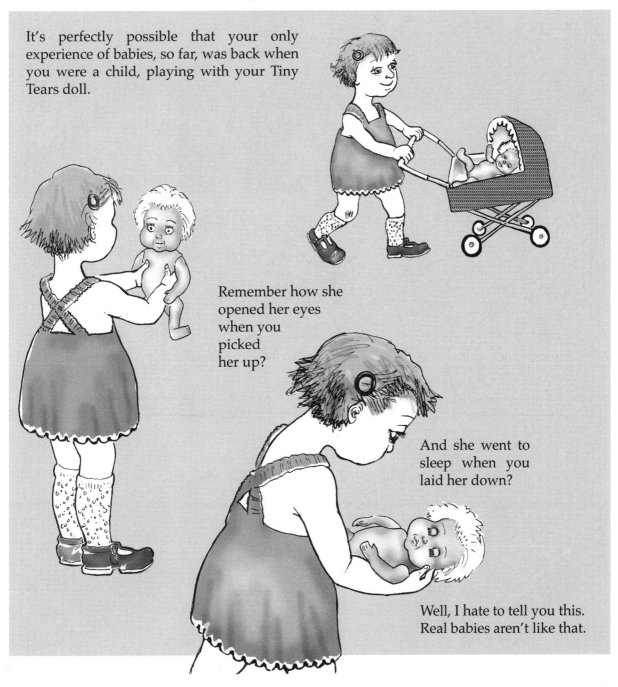

It's perfectly possible that your only experience of babies, so far, was back when you were a child, playing with your Tiny Tears doll.

Remember how she opened her eyes when you picked her up?

And she went to sleep when you laid her down?

Well, I hate to tell you this. Real babies aren't like that.

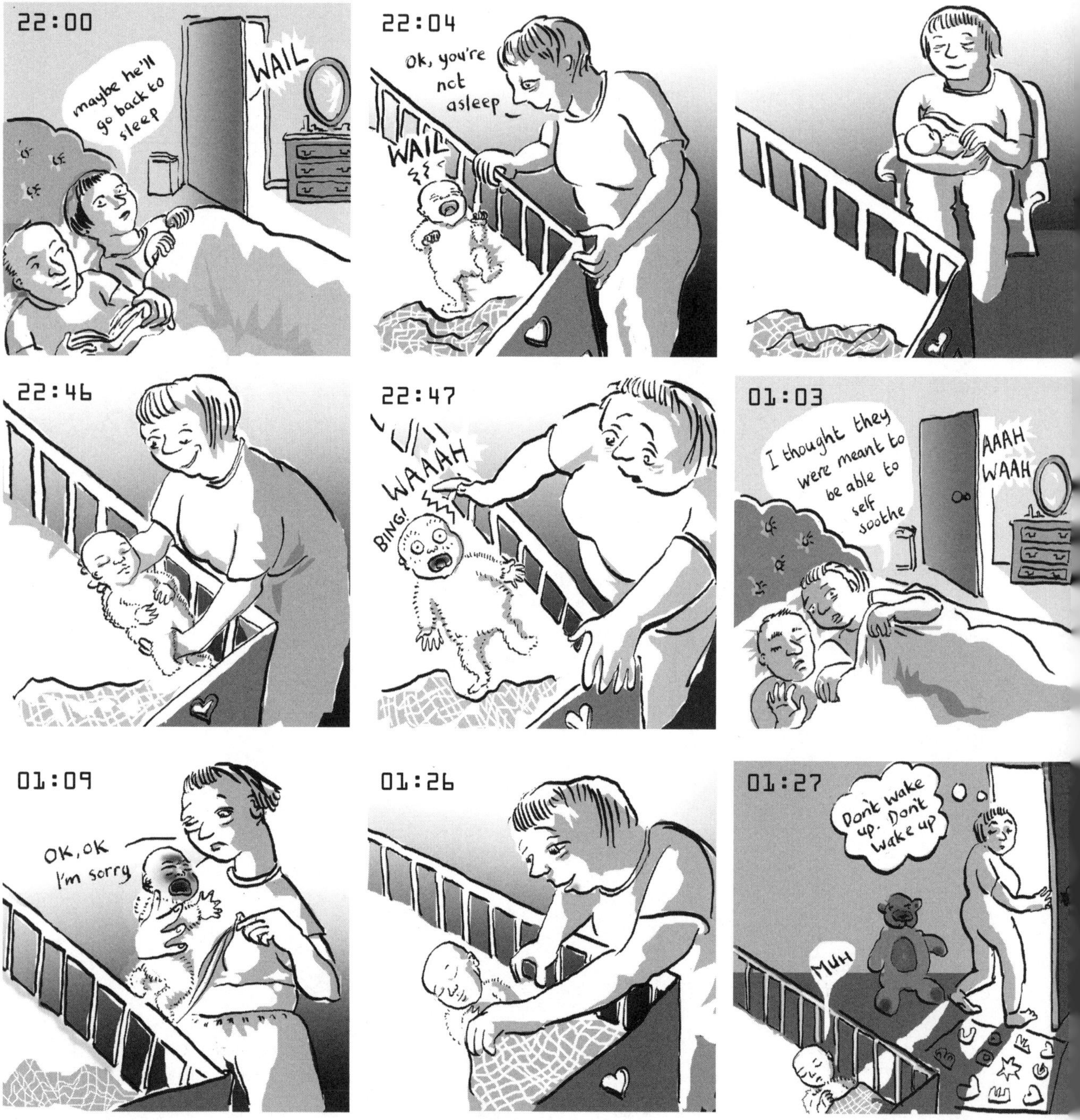
22:00
maybe he'll go back to sleep
WAIL
22:04
Ok, you're not asleep
WAIL
22:46
22:47
WAAAH
BING!
01:03
I thought they were meant to be able to self soothe
AAAH WAAH
01:09
OK, OK I'm sorry
01:26
01:27
Don't wake up. Don't wake up
MUH

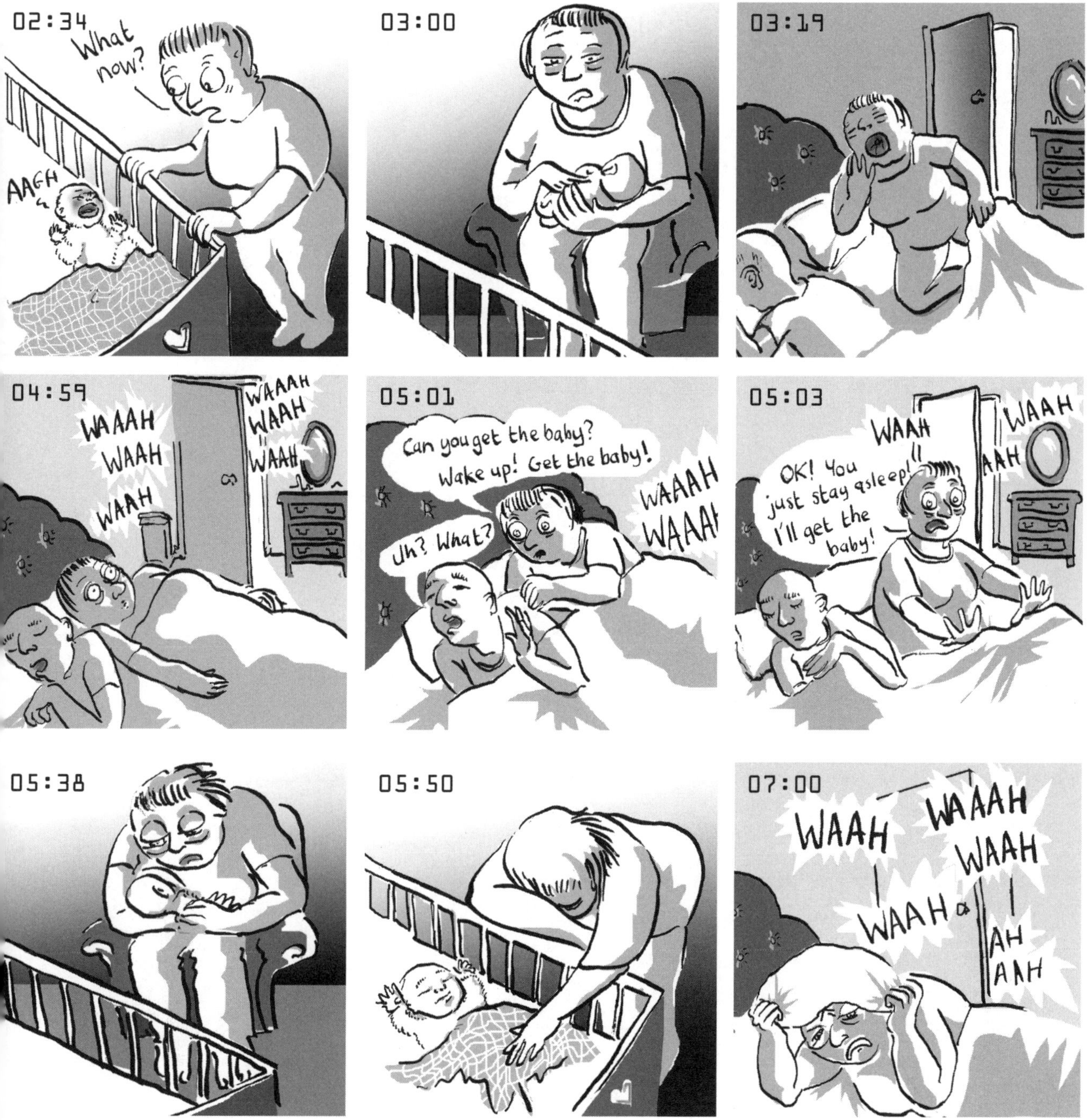
02:34
What now?
AAGH
03:00
03:19
04:59
WAAAH
WAAH
WAAH
WAAAH
WAAH
WAAH
05:01
Can you get the baby? Wake up! Get the baby!
Uh? What?
WAAAH
WAAA
05:03
OK! You just stay asleep! I'll get the baby!
WAAH
WAAH
05:38
05:50
07:00
WAAH
WAAAH
WAAH
WAAHa
AH
AAH

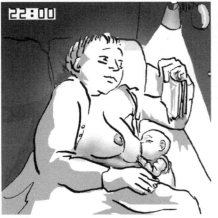
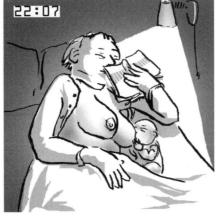
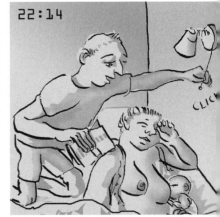
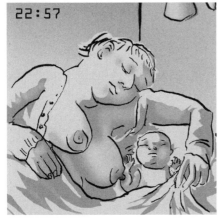
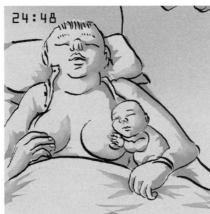
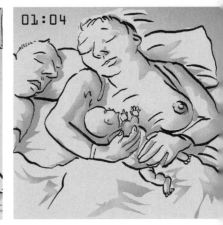
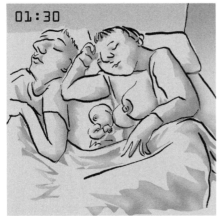
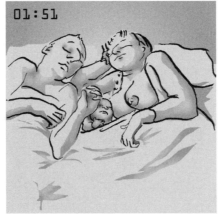
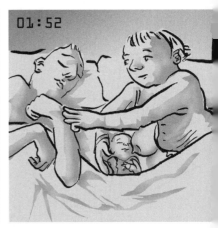

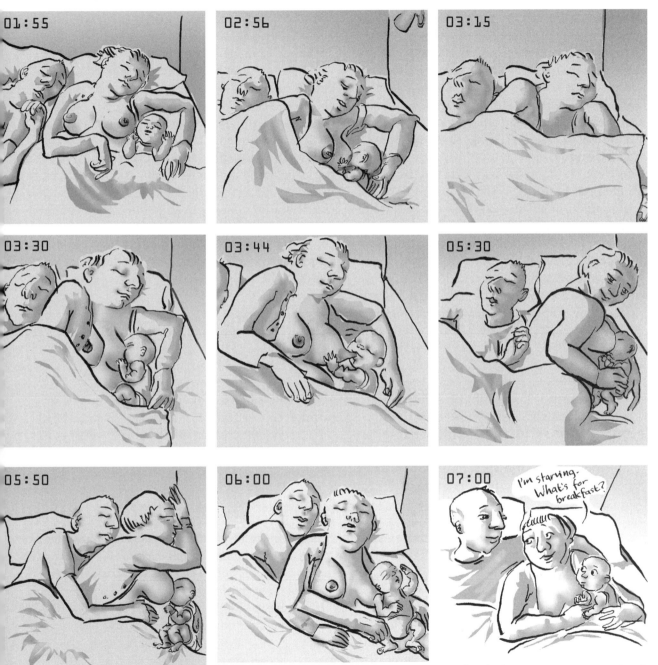

This mother is getting more sleep, and this baby is getting more food.

103

Of course, the main reason why most parents structure their time with their babies is so they can train them to sleep in cots. I never really saw the point in cots. My baby slept in my bed.

Now, a lot of the parenting books that I've read says that you should never bring your baby into your bed. They say, if you do, then your infant will develop 'lasting sleep problems'. Well, I disagree.

By the time my baby was four months old, I could come in from a walk, swing off the back carrier, tip him out, take off his snow suit, undo various layers of clothing, change his nappy, tuck him back together and lay him down on our bed. Without him waking up.

When he was two, his dad took him to a birthday party, and he fell asleep in the car on the way there. Soon after they arrived, it was time to cut the cake, and not wanting him to miss out, his dad tried to wake him up. And couldn't. That child was so damn good at sleeping that he didn't stir, even when suspended upside down by his ankles.

The sleep trainers will advise you to adopt certain measures to help your baby to go sleep in his own bed. Fit black-out blinds. Keep household noise to a minimum. Avoid eye contact when your baby is in her cot. The baby gets used to sleeping alone in the dark. But when a baby is always put to sleep in a darkened, quietened room, she'll be more easily startled awake by light or noise. And will grow up to be the adult who is kept awake at night by music from next door. This is so common in our society that we don't even see our light, disturbable sleeping habits as problematic.

If you'd seen my three-year-old son sound asleep on the sofa at my sister's twenty-first birthday party maybe you'd agree that he's got a robust, healthy ability to sleep through anything. Even her drunk friend sitting on him.

My son is now four. He didn't get his own bed until he was old enough to be enthusiastic about the idea. We still cuddle up together every night until he falls asleep and it generally takes about fifteen minutes. I spend quite a lot of time holding my child every evening, but not necessarily any longer than another parent might spend repeatedly packing their reluctant child back off upstairs to go to sleep on his own.

Babies and children gain reassurance from continued, loving human contact. Remember, there are tigers out there, and predators come out at night. I don't think my son has ever had a nightmare.

I just checked:

'Louie, have you ever had any dreams where it's horrible, and then you wake up?'

'No. I don't want one like that.'

Yet Gina Ford will tell you that night terrors are normal for cot-trained infants.

...parents find their child sitting bolt upright in bed screaming, eyes wide open and staring straight ahead as if witnessing something really horrific. Sometimes the screaming is accompanied by incoherent moaning and thrashing around, causing them to sweat so profusely that they appear to have a fever. Unlike the child who wakes up screaming after having a nightmare and looks for comfort and reassurance, a screaming child having a night terror cannot be comforted...

If I'm happy with my baby in my bed, why should anyone have a problem with that?

Why it's safe to sleep with your baby...

There are a lot of strong opinions on this sleeping issue. It's a common view in our society that it's dangerous and emotionally unhealthy for your baby to sleep in your bed. And there's a case to be made that it's dangerous and emotionally unhealthy for your baby to sleep in a cot in a nursery. Don't let anyone guilt trip you into making such a personal decision as where your baby sleeps according to what worked best for them. They're not you, and they don't know your baby.

You have a choice. But here is some information about co-sleeping (that is, sleeping with your baby), so it can be an informed choice.

Much of the fear that surrounds co-sleeping comes from an understandable apprehension that mothers will squash their babies in their sleep. But women have evolved to sleep with our babies, and we're actually very good at it.

Scientists have been videoing and monitoring co-sleeping mothers and babies to find out what it is that mothers do so well when they co-sleep. They found that women monitor their babies' temperature and position throughout the night, adjusting the blankets and checking them in their sleep. Many women learn to latch their babies on and feed them without coming fully awake.[1] In my experience, women also unconsciously monitor their babies' breathing. Once, my son's breathing became obstructed as he slept beside me. *I woke up.*

Mothers have an incredible capacity for monitoring their children which doesn't switch off at night. If you put your baby in a cot, even in your sleep you'll still have half an ear out for her cries. It's the same when you co-sleep, except that it's easier to put your hand on her to settle her when she wakes.

There is fear about babies dying in their sleep because it does happen. Sudden Infant Death Syndrome (SIDS) kills three hundred babies a year in the UK. No-one knows why. And so there has been a lot of research into cot death and whether co-sleeping is a causative or preventative factor.

Surprisingly, fewer babies die in countries where co-sleeping is common. In Beijing, more than half of all babies routinely sleep with their parents, and SIDS deaths are less than 0.01 per thousand. In Sweden, nearly half of all babies co-sleep and SIDS incidence is 0.02 per thousand. Here in the UK, the rate of sudden infant death is five times that.[2]

It could just be a genetic thing. Maybe white Western babies are more prone to cot death. After all, immigrant Bangladeshi mothers in the UK, who sleep with their babies (and who don't smoke) have SIDS rates far below the national average.[3] Yet the longer they live in the West, the more likely immigrants are to start using cots, whereupon their cot-death rates rise.[4]

So, could co-sleeping actually help protect against SIDS? Well, it's hard to be sure, because we don't know why SIDS happens, but there are indications that this could be the case.

Have you ever watched your little baby sleeping, and noticed how her breathing jerks in and out irregularly? Perhaps cot death happens when a baby simply forgets to breathe.

When a baby sleeps curled up by her mother, her breathing is more regular. As the mother breathes out, the carbon dioxide in her exhalation 'reminds' the baby to take another breath.[5] When babies sleep alone, the oxygen levels in their blood dip periodically. This doesn't happen when they sleep with their mums.[6]

Like adults, babies have different stages of sleep. There is the light, dream sleep where their eyes move and their faces twitch (so cute!), and there is the sound, heavy sleep where their limbs go floppy, and you know you can finally put them down. Unlike adults, babies have more light, dream sleep (which is when their brains do a lot of growing). Your husband might be able to crash out soundly and be snoring within minutes. Your baby will probably take a lot longer to settle.

It is during the second, heavy phase of sleep that cot death could be more likely to occur. Scientists have monitored babies who nearly died of cot death, but were resuscitated in time, and also the brothers and sisters of cot-death victims. They found that they moved less in their sleep than normal infants, woke up less in the night, and were more difficult to wake. If something obscured their breathing, they were less likely to struggle away. They were sleeping more deeply, which isn't necessarily healthy for a small baby.[7]

By contrast, when you put a baby in bed with her mother, she stirs more in her sleep, even during heavy sleep. Both the parent and the infant have more brief awakenings, where they don't become fully awake, they just touch base, and check each other are OK. The baby has more healthy light, dream sleep, and less potentially dangerous heavy sleep. Mother and baby wake together more of the time. Both mother and baby settle back to sleep quicker each time.[8]

Researchers have concluded that these brief awakenings protect babies against SIDS. Maybe trying to get small babies to sleep through the night on their own just isn't a very good idea.

Overheating is another known risk factor for cot death. Again, researchers have found that mothers monitor their babies during the night when they share a bed. They respond to changes in the room temperature and cover, or uncover, the baby accordingly. Although the babies do end up underneath the covers at times, the mothers shift and throw back the blankets in response. Co-sleeping babies have more stable temperatures than cot-sleeping babies.[9]

Babies are more at risk of SIDS if they sleep on their tummies. And babies sleep more on their tummies when they sleep in cots. Babies who sleep with their mothers curl up on their sides or their backs so they can keep snacking through the night.[10]

There has been no research into whether it is safe for a baby to go to sleep on her tummy, lying on your chest. It would seem to me, that if you have one of those babies who strongly prefers to lie on her front, then she would be best off lying on you, where you can monitor her breathing. Put her down on her back once she is fully asleep.

Co-sleeping is brilliant for breastfeeding, and breastfeeding helps protect against SIDS.[11] Babies get more than three times as many breastfeeds when they sleep with their mothers.[12] The breastfeeding hormone prolactin is higher at night. Frequent contact with the baby and the nipple boosts prolactin levels even higher, so you make better milk when you sleep with your baby.[13] I'd like to point out that if your baby does more of her feeding at night, while you are asleep, then she will need less feeding in the daytime, when you are awake and might rather be doing other things.

There is, however, one proven link between cot death and co-sleeping, and that is if you smoke. I'll say it again: *cigarettes are really bad*. When a mother sleeps and smokes in bed with her baby, the infant runs twelve times the risk of dying of SIDS.[14] Even when mothers don't smoke around their baby, the tar in their lungs means that they breathe out toxins that put the baby at risk. This skews the statistics. If you lump smoking mothers in with non-smoking mothers, then co-sleeping looks dangerous, when it isn't.[15]

'There is no evidence that bed sharing is hazardous for infants of parents who do not smoke.' That's a quote from the *British Medical Journal*. But occasionally babies do die of SIDS in bed with their parents, and society is quick to blame their bed sharing. The majority of babies die in cots, and no-one blames the cots.

Think about what else causes babies to die of cot death. Being poor is the biggest single risk factor.[16] You may not be able to do anything about that right now. Sleeping in a room with mould on the walls increases the risk.[17] Stress increases the risk.[18]

Sleeping in a separate bedroom increases the risk, and more UK cot deaths occur in a separate nursery than in anywhere else.[19] Really, don't bother decorating a nursery for your tiny baby. She'll be far more impressed if you wait until she's two. Whether your baby co-sleeps, or cot sleeps, let her sleep in the bedroom with you for the first year. Whether in the same bed, or in separate beds, mothers and babies are safest together.

The Rules

For co-sleeping to be safe, a mother's natural 'sleep alertness' should not be compromised. Don't co-sleep if you are drunk, or have taken sleeping tablets or other medications that 'may cause drowsiness'.

It is also recommended that you don't co-sleep when you are very tired. Ha ha ha. Very funny. How you are not meant to be very tired when you have a new baby is anyone's guess. However, the advice still stands, because very occasionally, a mother becomes so exhausted that she needs some very deep sleep away from her baby. If you hit a brick wall of exhaustion where it feels like your entire life is falling apart, then phone someone, anyone, to come and mind the baby while you get some sleep alone. This is yet another reason why new mothers need support. It's not a reason not to co-sleep.

The breastfeeding mother is the ideal co-sleeper. Your partner won't be as tuned in to the baby in the bed as you are. So for the first couple of months your baby is safer between you and the edge of the bed, with your partner on the other side. Always sleep like this if your partner smokes, and if he smells strongly of smoke, encourage him to shower and wash his hair before he gets into bed.

Make sure there is no risk of your baby suffocating or falling out of bed. Put your bed up against the wall, or sleep on a mattress on the floor. If you can't push your mattress flush with the wall, stuff the gap with folded blankets. Firm mattresses are best. If your mattress is soft and downy, you can put a thin camping mat under the sheet to make a firmer safe baby surface.

Keep the pillows away from the baby.

Free-flowing waterbeds are dangerous for babies to sleep on (the ones where you bob about like a ship at sea). 'Motionless' or 'fully stabilised' waterbeds are OK.

Don't wear dangly strings, longer than six inches, around your neck or off your nightclothes.

If you are really quite fat, as in, obese enough for it to affect your mobility, then your extra rolls of cuddliness might be too soft for your baby. If this is the case, you might want to try a co-sleeper, a crib that clips onto the side of your bed, so your baby still sleeps with you, but she has her own little zone.

You can make your own co-sleeper by taking one side off a conventional cot, bolting it to the side of your bed, and raising the mattress to the same height. (Again, fill any gap between the mattresses with firm rolled blankets.) This gives you 'baby area' and 'adult area', which you may be more comfortable with.

Never, ever sleep with your baby on a sofa. Or a beanbag. A remarkable number of babies die on sofas, because it's easy for the baby to become wedged between the cushions, and also because drunk people end up falling asleep on sofas with their babies.[20] You could consider replacing your sofa with a firm futon.

If you're staying at a friend's house and they offer you a sofa to sleep on, you can take all the cushions off, lay them on the floor, and tuck a blanket around them tightly to make a bed for you, and put the baby on the floor next to you on a folded blanket.

Don't let other children sleep next to the baby as they won't be sleep-alert like you. Put the baby between you and the wall, and practise feeding her off either breast (see page 103). Then you can let another child sleep on the other side of you if they need to.

Don't let pets sleep near the baby. I trusted my old dog to stay at the foot of the bed, but you might not want to risk that with your pet. And you might want the extra space.

Don't sleep with your baby if she has a disability that causes poor muscle tone.

Lay your baby to sleep on her back.

A word about overheating. Your baby is already wearing a nappy, you'll probably want to add a vest, and if scratchy toenails are a problem, a pair of socks. That's quite a lot of clothes. Quite apart from the safety issue, she's not going to be comfortable if she's too hot. Experiment with blankets to find an arrangement that works for you. You may want to use lighter weight bedding on the baby side of the bed. You might need to wear a cardigan to stop your neck and shoulders getting cold when you push the blankets away from the baby. You could put her in a fleecy sleep suit and keep her outside the blankets altogether.

If you bring the baby from a cot into your bed, you might need to take off a layer of her clothes.

Well, all that sounded extremely complicated didn't it? Basically it boils down to, don't sleep with your baby if you are drunk, drugged or if you smoke. Keep the baby away from soft things that might suffocate her, and unless you are very fat, that's not you.

You only need to set up your safe sleeping space once. Since practically everyone ends up sleeping holding their baby at some point, it makes sense to work out ahead of time where is a good safe zone (in your bed, away from the pillows) and where is dangerous (on the sofa, under the dog).

Why it's lovely to sleep with your baby...

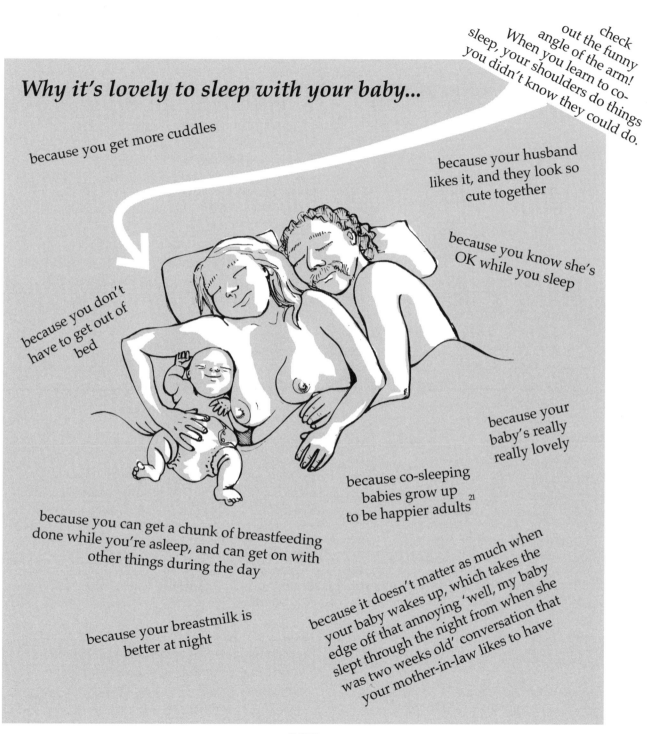

check out the funny angle of the arm! When you learn to co-sleep, your shoulders do things you didn't know they could do.

because you get more cuddles

because your husband likes it, and they look so cute together

because you know she's OK while you sleep

because you don't have to get out of bed

because your baby's really really lovely

because co-sleeping babies grow up to be happier adults [21]

because you can get a chunk of breastfeeding done while you're asleep, and can get on with other things during the day

because it doesn't matter as much when your baby wakes up, which takes the edge off that annoying 'well, my baby slept through the night from when she was two weeks old' conversation that your mother-in-law likes to have

because your breastmilk is better at night

Why it's really bloody annoying to sleep with your baby...

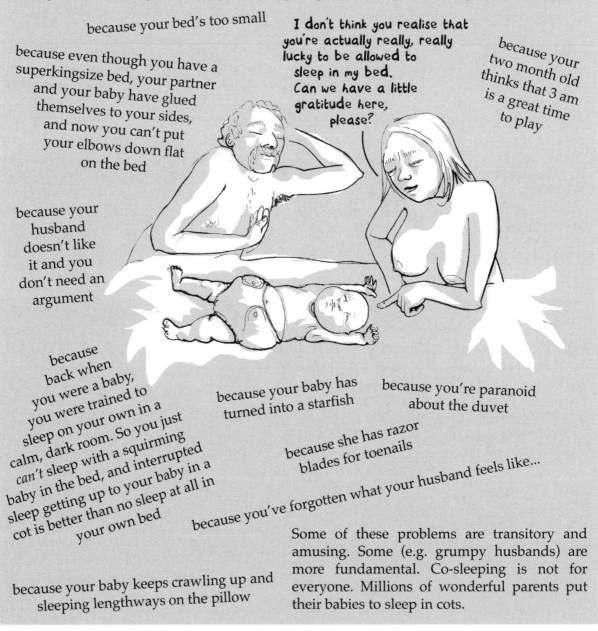

because your bed's too small

I don't think you realise that you're actually really, really lucky to be allowed to sleep in my bed. Can we have a little gratitude here, please?

because even though you have a superkingsize bed, your partner and your baby have glued themselves to your sides, and now you can't put your elbows down flat on the bed

because your two month old thinks that 3 am is a great time to play

because your husband doesn't like it and you don't need an argument

because back when you were a baby, you were trained to sleep on your own in a calm, dark room. So you just can't sleep with a squirming baby in the bed, and interrupted sleep getting up to your baby in a cot is better than no sleep at all in your own bed

because your baby has turned into a starfish

because you're paranoid about the duvet

because she has razor blades for toenails

because you've forgotten what your husband feels like...

because your baby keeps crawling up and sleeping lengthways on the pillow

Some of these problems are transitory and amusing. Some (e.g. grumpy husbands) are more fundamental. Co-sleeping is not for everyone. Millions of wonderful parents put their babies to sleep in cots.

Play it by ear...

Co-sleeping isn't the answer to everybody's sleep situation: it's a tool that parents can use safely to help them find their way. For me, it worked brilliantly. It went something like this: wake up, wriggle slightly, feed baby, both fall back to sleep. Repeat as necessary.

When he was three months old, my baby slept through the night. Just the once. I woke up at 7am with bosoms like barrage balloons, dripping milk everywhere. Ouch. Wake up child. Eat. I didn't want him to do that again in a hurry.

Gradually the spaces between the feeds became longer and longer. Now he always sleeps right through. But then, he is four years old, and has been weaned for some years.

Some babies are easier to sleep with than others. Some are lovely soft snuggly bundles. Some are manically wriggling energy balls. There are a few babies who are very 'sucky'. They like to fall asleep with the breast in the mouth, and then wake up if it isn't there. Childcare expert Martha Sears suggests placing your finger in her mouth and pressing firmly at the end of a feed to give her a secure feeling as you extricate yourself. Once your breastfeeding is well established, you can experiment with using dummies or helping her to suck her thumb. Or dad can hold her. Or you can find another solution that works for you.

Co-sleeping can take many forms. If you like, you can have a regular bedtime for your little one, where you bathe her and settle her in her cot and then get some special time with your partner. When she cries in the night you can bring her into your bed. You can use a cot as much as you want to, you don't have to be strict about it. You may find the sleep solution you have with one baby doesn't work so well with another.

Parents and kids can end up swapping between beds in co-sleeping households. Sometimes, your partner will really need some uninterrupted sleep, and may be better off sleeping elsewhere. My sister recounted a conversation she had with a friend that went something like this:

Friend: Oh, I'm ever so worried about Matthew having to sleep on the sofa while Noah is in your bed.

My sister: Matthew is thirty-four years old. I think that by that age my husband can cope with sleeping on his own for a few nights. He seems to be more rational and less needy than a seven-month-old baby.

You can experiment with the right time to move your baby out of your bed. Some babies will settle in a cot fairly easily – some are not so easily fooled.

I know a couple of mothers whose babies started out with them when they were tiny, and then, with some continuity and calm, settled in a cot when they were six months old.

I know a couple of mothers who sleep-trained their babies to a cot at a year, using the 'controlled crying' method. Try another book if you want to know about controlled crying, because I never had any truck with it. Waiting until a year seems to me to be a reasonable compromise on the sleep-training issue. If you are going to undertake a system of leaving your baby to cry to get used to her cot, then it would make sense to wait until she has built up a lot of loving trust with you and has some sense of cause and effect and the passage of time.

But if you're happy with her in your bed, you don't actually have to do the cot thing at all. At some point, you can sell the idea of having 'your own special bed like a big girl' to her. She'll probably quite like going to bed. It has always been nice for her so far.

If you don't do cots with your baby, you don't have to do bedtimes. She can fall asleep on you breastfeeding, and you can keep her with you until you go to bed. That's another personal thing. Some mothers really like to get their children all asleep by 7pm so then they can have some time off. But I work in the daytime, and I liked my baby to take long naps then, while I drew cartoons, so I could play with him in the evening. I also discovered that when my child goes to bed at 6.30pm, he wakes up at 6.30am. But if I don't put him down until 9pm, then I get more of a lie-in in the morning!

Co-sleeping seems to be parenting's best-kept secret. Studies in the US and the UK have shown that about a quarter of parents usually sleep with their babies, and more than two-thirds of parents sometimes do.[22] Incredible huh? That's quite likely to be you too, at some point, because sometimes babies just really, really want their mums.

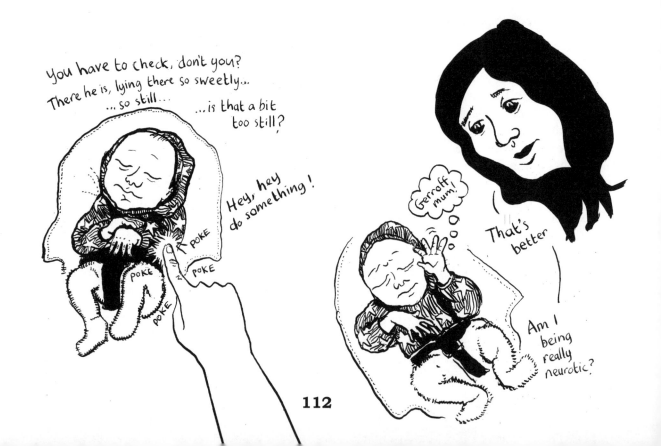

112

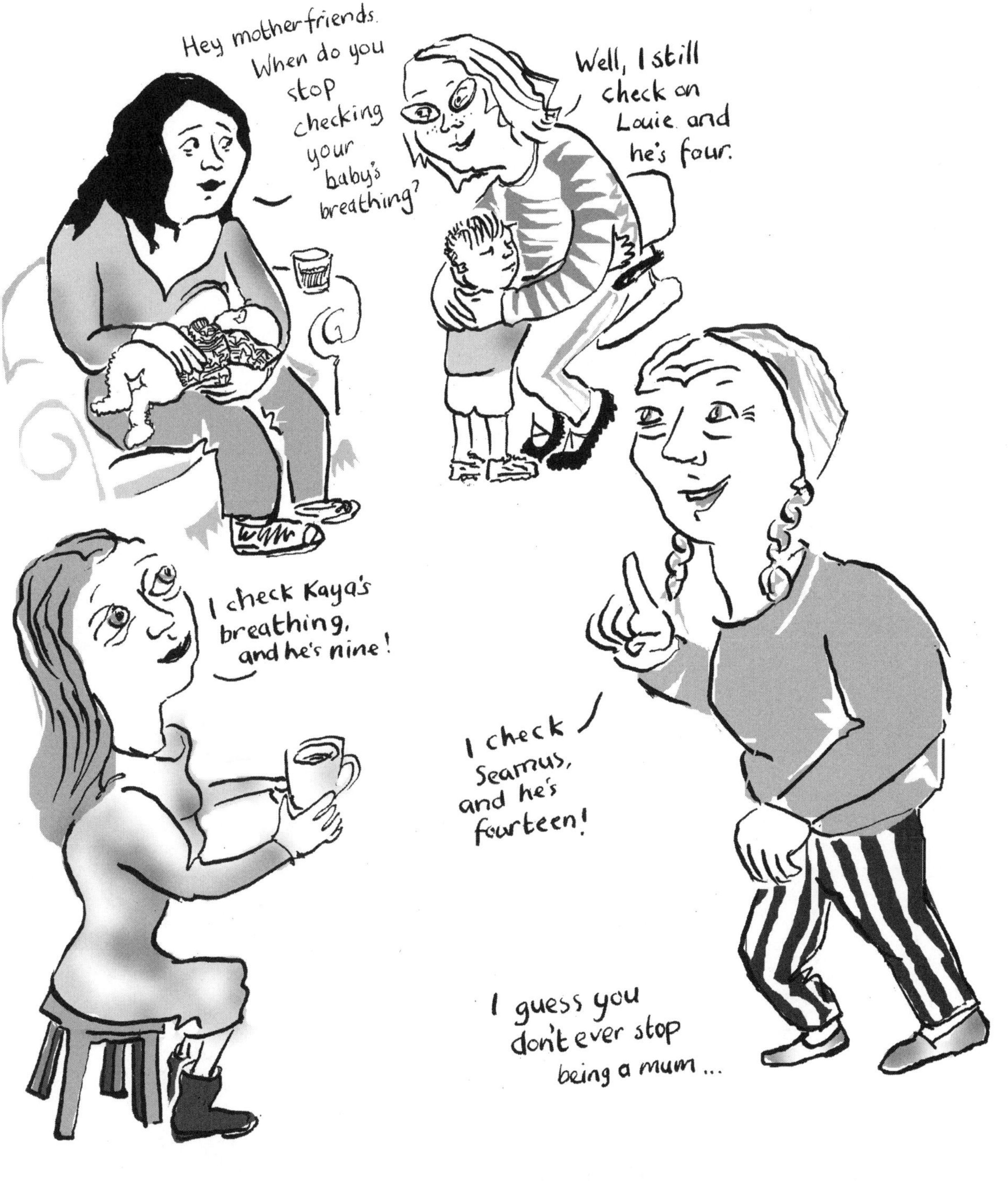
Hey mother-friends. When do you stop checking your baby's breathing?
Well, I still check on Louie and he's four.
I check Kaya's breathing, and he's nine!
I check Seamus, and he's fourteen!
I guess you don't ever stop being a mum...

Stress and depression

'You have a new baby?
That's WONDERFUL.'
'Oh, she's gorgeous. Lucky you!'
'You must be SO HAPPY.'

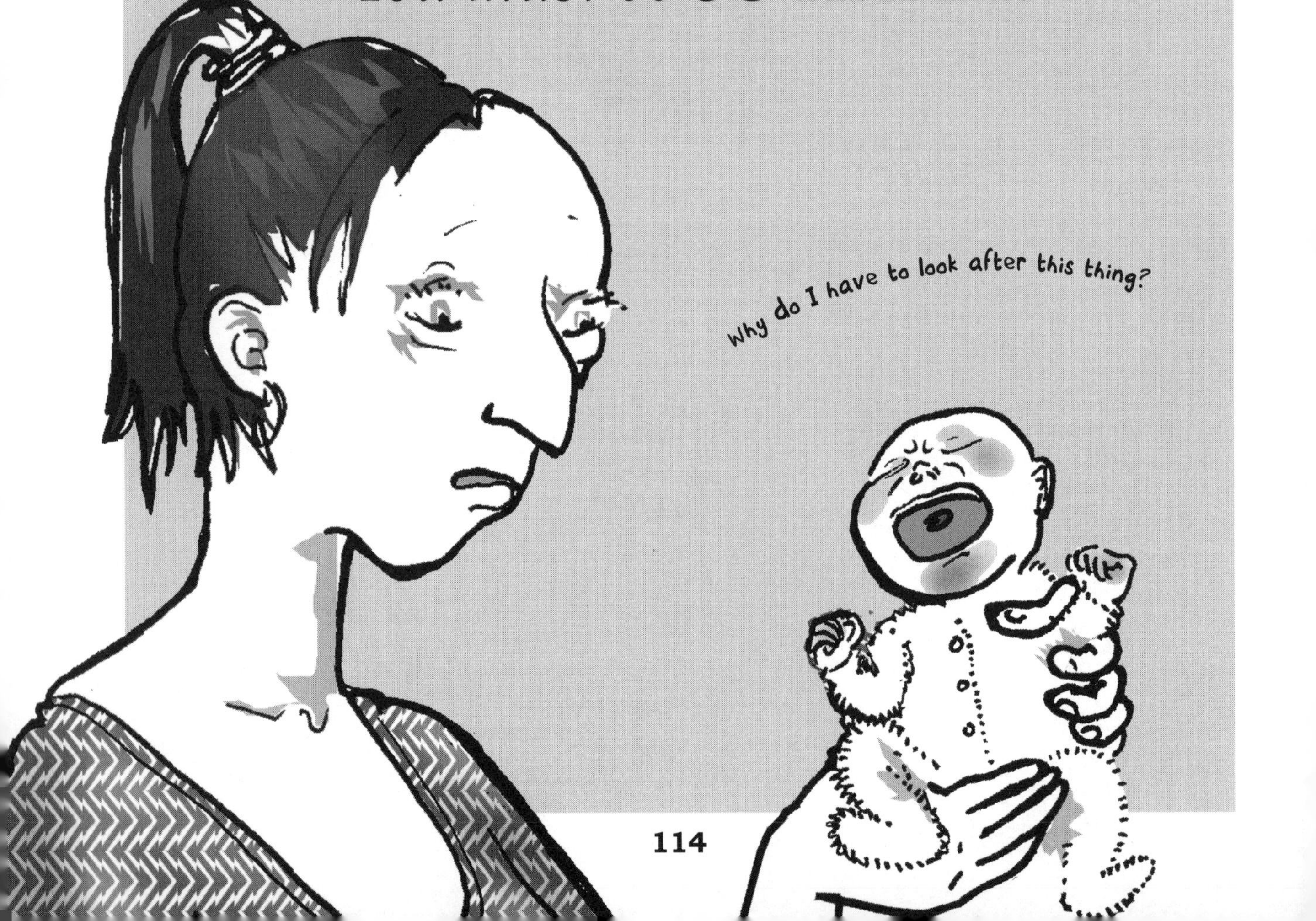

A quick brain chemistry lesson

The inner brain looks very similar in humans as in other animals. Your basic emotions are located here: fear, love, sexual desire. The inner brain also controls your hormone levels, your immune system, and other complicated and amazing things.

The outer level of your brain, the cerebral cortex, is packed full of logic circuits. A bit like a computer. It is much more highly developed in humans than in other animals, which is why we think we are so clever.

Actually, although the outer brain is good at processing information, it needs to work together with the basic feelings from the inner brain to be truly intelligent. If you don't have any sense of fear, or love, then you're not going to make sensible decisions.

Right in the centre of the middle of your brain is the amygdala, the 'seat of fear'. Should you be suddenly confronted by a rampaging panther when walking in the park, you wouldn't have time for your cerebral cortex to run through the logical outcomes of what might happen if you stick around. No, instead the amygdala takes over, triggering the fight or flight reflex: either you run for it, or you fight the panther off.

The amygdala tells the hypothalamus to get the body producing cortisol, the stress hormone. Cortisol is powerful stuff – it diverts all the body's energy to dealing with the threatening situation. Your immune system shuts down, so you're not wasting energy fighting disease. It switches off feelings of hunger, so you don't spend your energy eating or digesting. It makes you unable to relax, so you're hyped up to fight.

Your cerebral cortex, that is, your thought processes, stop working very effectively, narrowing things down into simple choices: stay here or run away.

The hippocampus (another important part of the inner brain, which deals with movement, learning and memory) is full of cortisol receptors. Once enough cortisol has been pumped out and these receptors are full, the hippocampus tells the hypothalamus to calm down. The danger has passed. Cortisol levels fall.

Sometimes this fight or flight reflex gets stuck. The receptors in the hippocampus get so overwhelmed that they don't work properly, cortisol floods the brain, the amygdala gets really excited (this must be a VERY BIG PANTHER!) and calls for more cortisol to ward off the danger. You are now seriously stressed. You become depressed.[1]

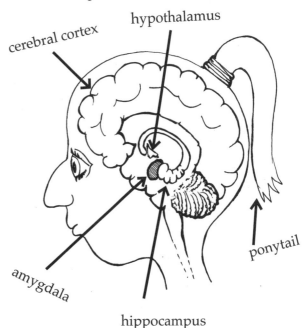

cerebral cortex

hypothalamus

amygdala

ponytail

hippocampus

Hey, did you think you were reading a book on breastfeeding? I already made you read about the social and political context of nineteenth-century childcare advice. Then we did developmental psychology. Now we're on to neurochemistry. I hope you're paying attention – there's more on cortisol and its role in human development later on in this chapter.

Depression is a normal part of human experience. It is also a common part of being a new mum. About half of new mothers feel tearful and radically unsure of themselves. One in ten women could be labelled as having 'clinical depression'.[2] Women from all walks of life get depressed. Queen Victoria had post-natal depression,[3] and she ruled the British Empire!

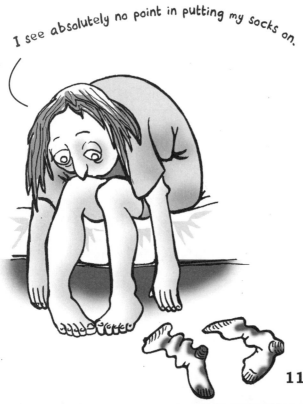

I see absolutely no point in putting my socks on.

Why do new mothers get depressed?

There are five things you need in order to be happy:

- A good diet.
- Plenty of exercise.
- The company of other people – laughter and touch are particularly important.
- Control over your life.
- Meaningful activity.

Knock out one of these five factors, and anyone can get depressed. Unsupported, mothers are vulnerable to all five:

- It is difficult to get the time to cook decent food.
- You can end up stuck in the house for days on end.
- All those people who used to be your best mates are off doing exciting things and all they ever talk about is work and all you can think about is nappies and rattles and teething gel and they don't understand and you're really boring and unsexy so maybe you should just stay in on your own
- …with this BABY, this incredibly NEEDY and VULNERABLE, wobbly-headed, dribbling person who wakes up every time you try to get something done and wakes you up every time you go to sleep.
- Meaningful activity? I haven't done anything all day. I haven't been ABLE to do anything all day. I haven't even done the housework. I'm just a mum.

116

Then what happens?

Well, the first thing that depression does is rob you of the ability to think objectively about your situation, and to do very much about it. As with all aspects of new mother support, it's far easier if someone else offers to help you, than if you have to ask for help. But I've already whinged about how bad it is that mothers are isolated, and blah, blah, we don't live in a perfect world. So here are some practical suggestions for helping to alleviate depression. And if you are reading this chapter and you're not depressed, maybe it will help you think creatively about how to help women who are.

Diet

Cortisol suppresses your appetite, so you don't feel hungry. So you don't eat a good diet. Which makes you more depressed. And you particularly need to eat regularly, now you are making all the food for someone else.

Most women have food issues. Being thin is so universally equated with being virtuous and desirable in the beauty culture of the modern media that it's hard not to feel some kind of triumph when you don't want to eat. Scrap that. Get yourself some easy, savoury, reasonably sustaining food (porridge is good) and eat a small portion of it every two hours throughout the day. It's going to help.

Sugar, on the other hand, doesn't help at all. Sweets give you a short, addictive burst of energy, followed by a physical and mental crash an hour later. These wild swings in your blood sugar don't help your mood. I'm sure that if you're craving sweets and cakes for comfort, me telling you that you're not allowed them isn't going to make you any happier. So I'm not going to do that. I do recommend that you think about savoury foods that you like, and increase the amount of those you eat instead. Don't worry about getting fat right now. Concentrate on getting happy.

Exercise

All the cortisol that is racing round your body, bizarrely, robs you of energy. Because your stress hormones are on permanently, you can't relax properly, and may find it very hard to fall asleep. Which isn't great, when you're about to be woken up in two hours anyway. When you do sleep, your brain races around in uneasy, repetitive dreams, trying to 'solve' the Massive Panther that is stalking your psyche. Which is why you wake up feeling like a zombie, and your thought processes are so stupid all day. (Although everyone with a new baby feels like a zombie anyway because getting woken every two hours isn't funny in itself.)

It's going to take a big effort for you to do any exercise. Even if you're not depressed, leaving the house with a small baby is a bewilderingly complicated exercise that can take over an hour to accomplish. If you've had no refreshing sleep at all, then it can seem impossible. Still, you need to do it. Strap your baby into a sling and walk somewhere. It doesn't matter where. If you can talk to someone while you're out as well, even if it's just a daily chat with the lady in the paper shop, then that's good. Carrying your baby keeps her warm, keeps you both close, increases the exercise you're getting and, if it's a good sling, means you can feed her on the go.

If you can arrange a babysitter, you could go swimming, or to an exercise class such as yoga or tai chi.

Social interaction

Now this is a big one. Say your husband just spent his paternity leave down the pub; no-one came round to look after you for your confinement; the relatives have all departed leaving you several dubious outfits for the baby and a heap of contradictory advice. Just who are you meant to hang out with?

It will help you prevent depression from setting in if you stay in touch with the women from your antenatal classes. The National Childbirth Trust and the La Leche League may all run mothers meetings in your area. Baby swimming, massage or signing classes are another way to meet other mums. The Meet-a-Mum Association has been set up specifically to help mothers who are feeling depressed to find supportive friends. Internet chat rooms are another good way to socialise with other mothers, as are texting and phoning your friends.

Once you are depressed, you may feel like you can't face seeing other people. Those crazy, distorted thought processes really don't help you reach out to other people. Everything is black or white; either/or. You can no longer appreciate the complexities of human interaction. You can't see the shades of grey.

'She said she couldn't meet up tomorrow THEREFORE she doesn't like me.'

'My baby is crying THEREFORE I am a bad mother.'

'Her baby is not crying THEREFORE she is a good mother, and it's all fine and easy for her.'

'They are all good mothers THEREFORE they will laugh at and judge a bad mother like me'.

'Billions of women have had babies before me THEREFORE it must be a really easy job THEREFORE I must be very stupid and bad to be finding it so difficult.'

Spending time with other people helps because it snaps you out of the negative thoughts that circle round and round and round your head. It can be good to get involved in other people's lives and discover that they have troubles too. Meeting up with other mothers, you'll discover that no-one's finding it easy. The sympathetic companionship of other people who know what it's like can be a soothing balm to your raw nerves.

Sometimes you might find that you can't tell friends and social acquaintances how you are feeling. Cortisol is so powerful that it blocks out loving feelings. It interferes with the prolactin and oxytocin that you get when you're with your baby. You may be wondering what on earth I'm going on about when I refer to breastfeeding as a pleasant experience, and to babies as wonderful and amazing. That might not be what it's like for you. You might feel a flat nothing, or even hatred for your baby. That's a logical position for a mother who is experiencing extreme stress.

Hallucinations can also accompany depression. This is normal. If you put anyone under enough stress, they will experience voices or visions. Many cultures channel this extraordinary human ability, and use fasting and sleep deprivation to induce shamanic experiences. Very religious people often experience pleasant, controlled hallucinations. Sitting in on your own in a flat with a crying baby, hearing voices and thinking that you're going mad is neither pleasant nor controlled.

Bursts of manic energy, where you feel great, yet entirely disconnected from life are another sign that your brain chemistry isn't right, and that you must get some help.

Talk to your health visitor, your midwife or your GP, phone the Association for Postnatal Illness or the Samaritans. All these people know that your situation is common. They are not going to take your baby away from you. Nothing that you have to say will shock them. Talking openly about how you are feeling is the simplest cure for stress known to humankind.

The worst example of muddled thinking that goes with depression is the urge to kill yourself. 'Life is awful, therefore I would be better off dead. No-one would miss me.' Suicide is not a sensible option here. It is a permanent solution to a temporary condition. People get better from depression every day; it just doesn't feel like that when you're depressed. I appreciate that this is a difficult situation, but dammit girl, you don't want to suddenly realise that you had loads of friends all along when they turn up to your funeral.

It is always worth asking a depressed person if they have thought of suicide. Then ask them if they have a plan for how they would go about it. If you talk openly about the subject then you are in a position to point out the flaws in their argument, ie you *would* really miss them a *lot*. Sit down and make a list with them. Draw a line down the middle of a piece of paper, and put the reasons for killing yourself on one side, and the reasons for not killing yourself on the other side. Make the second list longer than the first, and write it in bigger letters. Your friend's capacity for logic is working on a very simple level here, so she'll find this convincing.

Try not to be dismissive when a friend confides to you that she is finding life difficult. Ask her more about how she feels.

Here's another good tip for interacting with someone who is depressed, even if they are suffering from extreme trauma. Get them on their own. Make them a cup of tea and encourage them to talk about what is upsetting them. Then, very simply ask them 'what is the worst thing about your situation?' Listen to them. Then ask them 'what can you do to make that better?' You can help anyone access their inner resources with just these two simple phrases.[4]

That is not to say that every conversation you have with a depressed person has to revolve around how awful they are feeling. Once you have discussed the issues openly, and helped your friend to improve her situation, you can also help distract her from negative thoughts. Acknowledge her mood, then help her shift it by doing something together that you both enjoy.

Control over your life

Another big one. Having a baby represents a massive loss of control over your life. You might have planned and wanted a baby for years, or your first baby might be the result of an unexpected contraceptive slip-up. In either case, you didn't expect it to be quite like this. The old, child-free you has completely gone. No matter what happens now, you will always be this new person, a mother, which is a reason to celebrate, but also, maybe, to mourn.

If you are prepared for the realities of childrearing it will come as less of a shock. The modern culture of childcare instills some pretty unrealistic expectations in new parents. No, your baby probably isn't going to sleep through the night. And the chances are that she will want to feed more often than every four hours. She is going to need a lot of you. She's going to push you to give more than any one person can. If you want to, you can try and modify all these behaviours, sensitively, and over time. But don't expect them to not be there in the first place.

Have a look at other areas of your life which may be out of control.

How was the birth of your baby? It almost certainly wasn't the way you imagined it would be. No matter how hard you study all the options open to you when you write your birth plan, babies very rarely arrive according to the script. It is good that the natural birth movement exists to help women achieve a goal of unmedicated labour, but that doesn't mean that every baby can or should be born without medical intervention. *Some babies need to be born by Caesarean*. This may leave you grieving for the natural labour that you planned. The home birth pictures on pages 62 to 65 might make you feel upset.

Distressing birth experiences often occur when a woman is unsupported in labour, with birth attendants who undermine her choices for no good reason. If that happened to you, you have a right to be angry. It would be helpful if more hospitals adopted a policy of encouraging mothers to give feedback on negative birth experiences.

However, even if the birth was, overall, a good one, a small detail may be significant to you: the fact that you weren't allowed to hold your baby straight away, or the attitude of a doctor present. You don't have to be obsessive about this, but you are allowed to be upset.

Writing an account of the birth will help. Maybe the purpose of the weepy 'baby blues' that happens a few days after the birth is to help you to acknowledge this massive event, and the fact that it can be both happy and also, very scary.

Your need for a stable, secure home increases when you have a child. Were you forced to move house during pregnancy? Are you currently happy with where you are living? If not, can you move?

Has a loved one died? Grief is a massive stress. Don't expect too much of yourself. It's going to hurt. Remember that the dead person would want you to be able to carry on with life. Don't feel you are betraying them by dedicating yourself to the living. Free specialist bereavement counselling is available through CRUSE.

Are you grieving for a previous child, stillbirth, miscarriage or abortion? Feelings of guilt can interfere with your bond with the new baby. It is common to feel that this new baby shouldn't be here, and to wish for the old one back. Anger is part of grief. But this living baby needs you too, and your bond with her will get better with time. Writing to or about your previous child, or making a scrapbook of memories can help with the grieving process.

If there a particular friend or relative who is being subtly unhelpful? You can decide to break off contact with someone for a time so you can concentrate on your own emotional needs.

How is your relationship with your partner? If it isn't good, can you both attend counselling to try and improve it? If it is very bad, do you need to split up? If it is at all violent, contact your local women's refuge for help.

What was your childhood like? Was that horribly out of control?

Now you are suddenly a parent yourself, and you are responsible for a tiny, vulnerable baby. What if the tiny, vulnerable baby that you once were was never properly mothered? You are going to find it difficult to deal with the needs of another, if your basic needs were never met.

Parents are all-powerful to children. They are beyond criticism. Children have a psychological need to love their parents unquestioningly. When parents mess up, children blame themselves. This is less scary than blaming the parent, their only means of survival.

There may have been trauma in your childhood, physical or sexual abuse, loss or grief which you have not had a chance to think about until now. You may have been keeping busy, developing coping strategies, rationalising that everything is OK. Now you have undergone a major life change, and you're trying to construct your own family. You need to come to terms with where your childhood went wrong and the fact that you were not to blame.

Then again, there may have not been any specifically terrible events which blighted your childhood. There may just have been a continual stream of negative criticism. This is very common in our society, and it's really destructive. If you tell a small child that she's a bad person, then she will believe it. If that small child was you, then get help now. Otherwise you may find yourself reflecting your frustrations back onto your child. You can break this cycle.

The good thing about unhappy childhoods is that they don't have to translate into unhappy adulthoods. There are plenty of happy, well-adjusted people out there who had hellish childhoods. If you can go over events (generally with someone else) and work out what happened, and maybe why it happened, and acknowledge your childhood feelings, then you can start to move on.

Meaningful activity

Looking after a baby is meaningful activity, but our society doesn't reward it with very high status. Motherhood is work, but you don't get paid, you don't get *any* time off, it's really difficult to see your day-to-day achievements and most of what women do goes completely unrecognised, even by themselves.

Psychotherapist Naomi Stadlen has filled a book with descriptions of all the vital tasks that mothers do that we don't even have words for (*What Mothers Do* – it's a really good read). If we don't have words for it, how can we evaluate just what it is that we're doing? If you view yourself as someone who isn't even managing to be a housewife, you'll have a pretty low opinion of your abilities. If, instead, you recognise that you are being the primary support system for the next generation, responsible for the continuance of the human race, you might start to feel more appropriately proud of your broken nights' sleep. Really, we deserve medals, we do.

When you are depressed, you can miss out on the love hormones that keep mothers going. If you don't get the positive rewards of prolactin and oxytocin, your job is extra difficult. Many mothers get depressed yet still keep a good, loving connection with their babies. But some women are under so much stress that their relationship with their babies breaks down. The baby ends up crying more and becoming needier. This vicious circle can be broken with rest, love and support.

And depressed women may be more likely to have difficult babies. Cortisol passes through the placenta, so stressful events in pregnancy or a difficult forceps birth can result in babies that are more difficult to soothe. Alcohol abuse or smoking in pregnancy can also make a baby jumpy. These babies need more continuous contact and more frequent feeds than their placid, unstressed peers.[5]

Sorry, didn't mean to depress you there.

In my experience, when I was upset and at the end of my tether, my baby cried more. When you're crying inside, then your baby's screams sound right to you. It's like he's expressing something that you can't give voice to yourself.

There is also an element of chicken and egg about this. There are some babies who just cry a lot when they are very young. These mothers really do need support. Holding an unsoothable baby while he screams for hours is a soul-destroying experience that is bound to make any mother depressed.

So here's some more help...

Drug therapy is a good option for many

people with depression, and can work very well to help you out of a difficult place. The older tricyclic antidepressants are safe for use while breastfeeding. You will need to take your antidepressant for several months, at least, and it may be a few weeks before you first feel the full benefit. Stay in regular touch with your GP to monitor your improvement, and talk to her about reducing the dose gradually when you are ready to come off it. A small trace of the drug you are taking will pass into your milk, but your breastmilk is still better for your baby than formula, so don't feel guilty about that.

If you find that the drugs you are taking are making things worse, particularly if you start to suffer from uncontrollable urges or suicidal thoughts, then go back to the doctor straight away. The drug may need to be changed.

Unfortunately, the newer SSRI drugs like Prozac have never been tested on breastfeeding women, and are not licensed for use by them. This can lead to a situation where depressed women are pressured to stop breastfeeding in order to take a more effective antidepressant medication. In this case, consider your options carefully.

If breastfeeding is going well, then being forced to stop now may make your depression worse.[6] Breastfeeding hormones actually help you to feel happy, and feeding your baby can help you feel close. SSRI drugs don't necessarily work well for everyone. There are other effective strategies you can use, and other drugs you can take.

If breastfeeding is difficult, but you really want it to succeed, then giving up at this point may make you feel like a failure. Contact a lactation consultant for help with your breastfeeding problems. She will enjoy helping you. It's her job.

But if you have tried breastfeeding and you don't like doing it then wean! It's the twenty-first century! You have a choice! See page 184 for help with weaning strategies. Also, if you have used SSRIs before and you know that they work well for you, then stopping breastfeeding and starting medication can be a positive choice that will improve your parenting and make you and your baby happier.

Stop taking the *contraceptive pill* or mini-Pill. The Association for Postnatal Illness advise that it may be making your depression worse. You can discuss other contraceptive options with your GP or health visitor.

Try *acupuncture* or *shiatsu*. Chinese medicine sees illness, whether physical or mental, as the result of deficiencies in the energy flows passing around the body. Having a baby takes a lot out of you, so it's not surprising if your 'vital force' is running low. It's nice to have such a simple, non-judgmental explanation for why you might be feeling completely insane. Acupuncture works.[7]

St John's Wort is a herbal remedy which is proven to work against depression.[8] You can buy the tincture, also known as Hypericum, at healthfood shops and some chemists. Take the dose recommended on the bottle. This is easy to do at the first signs of depression. Like conventional antidepressants, it takes a few weeks to feel the full benefits from St John's Wort. Wean yourself off the dose gradually.

You can't use St John's Wort if you are taking other antidepressants, the contraceptive pill or the prescription drugs loperamide, cyclosporin, amitriptyline, digoxin, indinavir, warfarin, phenprocoumon or theophylline,[9] but you can consult a medicinal herbalist for more treatment options.

Fish oil supplements and evening primrose oil actually strengthen your brain.[10]

Massage helps for depression.

Counselling will help if there are issues to do with your own parenting that you wish to explore. Counselling is available on the NHS, but there may be a waiting list.

Cognitive behaviour therapy

is as beneficial for depression as any drug.[11] It helps you change patterns of negative thinking and boosts your self-esteem. You can get good results quite quickly, and you don't have to trawl over distressing episodes from your past. Private practitioners sometimes offer it in conjunction with hypnotherapy. You may be able to get cognitive behaviour therapy on the NHS. There are also CD-roms and free internet-based resources that you can access.

Time away from your baby.

If the strain of motherhood has got to you to such an extent that it's affecting your mental health, you need some support. Find a friend, ask a relative, employ a childminder, do what it takes to get some regular respite so that you can get some sleep and concentrate on yourself for a while. Don't feel you have to rush around getting things done during this time, unless you want to.

Time with your baby.

Work on your bond with your baby. Spend time cuddling and relaxing and bathing together. Baby massage is excellent for helping you connect with each other. Singing will help your depression and babies love singing – fortunately, they don't care at all if it is completely out of tune! Go out to baby activities if you want. If you can afford it, consider getting someone in to clean the house so you can concentrate on your child.

Many women don't start off with an instant

bond with their babies. It's like falling in love with anyone – for some people it happens at first sight, while other people find that their feelings build more gradually. They are all brilliant mothers.

Depression is a serious condition. All these strategies, as well as improved diet and exercise, need to be done regularly to see results.

Another brain chemistry lesson

Thanks to the wonders of magnetic resonance imaging (MRI scanners), scientists are now able to study what is going on in living thinking brains. This is a lot more informative than dissecting dead ones. And the discovery that the stress hormone cortisol can be detected in swabs of saliva (easier to collect than blood samples) means that psychologists now have an exact way of measuring how and why people get stressed, even when they are very young babies.

Our second neurochemistry lesson is based on the book *Why Love Matters* by Sue Gerhardt which is an overview of recent discoveries about babies and stress. I advise you to read it. For a book about human psychology it's pretty accessible. However, you've just had a baby, you may be somewhat short of sleep and your powers of concentration may not be at their highest. So here's my attempt to describe Gerhardt's conclusions using shorter words.

All babies are born with a unique personality. Some are quick to anger; others are easy to please. But it's a baby's relationship with his loving carers in his early years that to a large extent determines how that personality will turn out.[12] This 'unrememberable and unforgettable'* period sets the benchmark for how he will deal with his emotions in later life.

Because babies are so helpless, they need constant maintenance. Thinking about it from the baby's point of view, every day presents a thousand different ways to get stressed. Hungry? Have to cry. Tired? Have to cry. Got your toe stuck in a blanket? Cry.

What the baby's carer does is continually soothe the stresses from the baby's existence. A baby can't soothe himself – you have to do it for him. The amazing thing is that every time you do it, you're setting him up to be able to deal with stress effectively his whole life long.

Stress for babies works just the same way as it does for adults. The amygdala prompts the hypothalamus to get cortisol production going. Cortisol receptors in the hippocampus fill up and the hippocampus feeds back to the hypothalamus the information that we've got enough cortisol now, thank you very much, and we don't need any more.

Babies and children who are cuddled and held lots and given plenty of positive attention grow into adults who have lots of cortisol receptors in the hippocampus. This means they are better able to cope with stressful events in their life, and are less likely to become depressed.[13]

On the flip side, if a baby is frequently left in a state of stress for long periods of time then that cortisol stays whizzing around their system. The cortisol receptors in the hippocampus get overwhelmed and shut down. Because young babies' brains are still forming, this can have a lasting effect; they end up with fewer cortisol receptors and may always be more prone to

* this phrase is by psychoanalyst Alvin Frank.

stress and depression.[14] Children who had very stressful babyhoods tend to either be consumed by anxiety (ambivalent attachment) or they learn to switch their stress response off (avoidantly attached).[15] Because cortisol suppresses the immune system, they are also more likely to be ill.[16]

A baby's brain grows at an amazing rate in the first year – it more than doubles in weight.[17] Connections start firing up between all the neurons in the brain, and patterns start to form. The brain starts to register experiences which are repeated and familiar, and they become expected, they feel 'right' to the child. Even if they aren't very nice.[18]

So a baby whose mother reacts to him with pleasure and delight will seek out positive relationships in later life. But babies whose mothers are hostile and rejecting can go on to repeat the trauma with abusive partners. Somehow the unpleasant behaviour just makes sense to them. This fundamental link between early experience and adult behaviour explains a lot. Like why my friend Paul, who was beaten as a small child, somehow never could leave a party without getting punched.

There is a whole section of the brain that hardly even starts developing until after the baby is born. This is the front brain and especially a part of it called the orbitofrontal cortex.[19] Remember how the brain is divided into the inner emotional part and the outer logic-processing section? Well the orbitofrontal cortex joins the two together. It's where you learn to think about your emotions. It helps you identify with others, and empathise with them. When it develops well, it enables you to use your logical brain to temper feelings of lust, or rage or shame, and display appropriate behaviour in a given social setting. I think we all know people whose orbitofrontal cortexes don't quite work as well as they should.

On the extreme end of the child abuse spectrum, scientists have studied Romanian orphans who were tied into their cots as babies, fed, watered and ignored. Some of them never really developed orbitofrontal cortexes and have extreme difficulty regulating their emotions.[20]

But most babies have mothers. Mothers naturally help their babies learn to name what they are experiencing. 'Oh, you're hungry,' 'you're tired,' 'that's scratchy, isn't it?' 'look, there's an elephant!' – those repetitive conversations that sound so mundane when you haven't got a baby, yet are so absorbing when you have, are vitally important. By naming the child's emotional state, the mother helps him to get in touch with his feelings. Soothing your baby and giving him lots of positive feedback actually creates his good, working orbitofrontal cortex.

The other amazing thing about baby's brains is that cuddles help them grow. Smiles, and reassuring touches trigger off the release of the natural happy-chemical beta-endorphin and the neurotransmitter dopamine. These biochemicals actually help the brain, particularly the front brain, to develop. So there's no need to plonk your baby in front of a Baby Swot DVD – having lots of lovely snuggles will make him more clever.[21]

There is an obvious conclusion that can be drawn, that you don't need a PhD in neuroscience to come up with. If you love your children, and listen to them, then you set them up to be loving, listening children in turn.

Reading all this might just make you feel paranoid, guilty and scared that you're going to give your baby brain damage. What exactly are you meant to do with this information?

Babies do get stressed, and babies cry. If, while you listen to her, you start wondering whether her baseline cortisol levels are going fundamentally awry, then that's going to make you even more upset. Which will in turn make her more upset.

The scientists say that babies need lots of cuddles to make them clever. And the sleep-training experts say that babies need lots of sleep to make them clever. And there are many loving, considerate parents who aren't getting more than two hours of unbroken sleep at a time, who need some practical advice on what to do about it.

The first advice that many parents are given is to leave the baby to cry it out. Controlled crying sleep modification programmes are based on the idea that you leave your baby in a cot to cry, but that you check on her at intervals without taking her out of the cot. After a couple of nights of heart-rending tears, the baby gets the idea that the cot is the place to go to sleep and she settles down for longer stretches. It can be effective, but is it safe?

The science indicates that base levels of cortisol are still being set in the first six months of life,[22] so I would infer that leaving your child alone to cry in this period is potentially harmful. That is not to say that every young baby who undergoes controlled crying ends up as a depressive wreck – a lot depends on a child's temperament and on other factors – but if you look at the scientific mechanisms involved, it's probably not a good idea.

By a year, the cortisol regulation system has settled down, so a well-socialised baby won't produce dangerous levels of stress hormones when he is upset.[23] If you can hold out well past six months and preferably until your baby is over a year old, then that's a more developmentally appropriate age to sleep train. Choose the gentlest method on offer. It's only OK if it works. Some children will resist sleep training, so give up with them and try something else. There are books with alternatives to controlled crying listed on page 196.

But it's worth bearing in mind that when a loving parent does an episode of sleep training, we're talking about a short period of crying in an otherwise functional relationship, and that's unlikely to have lasting ill effects. The babies who suffer are the ones whose parents are consistently neglectful, usually because they are so distanced from their own emotions that they find it very difficult to regulate someone else's.

You see, when it comes to childcare, there are a lot of different ways of doing it right.

The style of babycare that I used with my son is, I have since discovered, known as attachment parenting. Check it out on the internet. There are loads of websites about it, and I think it's great. But, you know what? It's a style, not a prescription.

I mean, I really like my child to wear granny's hand-knitted jumper. Other mothers would quietly consign it to the bottom drawer. I have always favoured wooden toys for children. Other parents prefer plastic, noisy toys. All the babies I've ever met just love plastic noisy toys, so they probably have a point. I have a horror of the sweatshop economy, so prefer to buy second-hand things for my son (an area of my life where ethical considerations dovetail nicely with financial necessity). Other parents scrimp and save so that they can get a new pushchair for their child, as a symbol of giving them a good start in life. None of that has anything to do with how happy your baby is.

The co-sleeping, drag 'em around and breastfeed 'em anywhere thing doesn't work with every baby. Children who are on the autism/Asperger's spectrum need regularity and routine – they'll never cope very well with Spanish fiestas. My amazing baby nephew Alfie has Down's syndrome – it's not safe for him to sleep in an adult bed, and he does very well in a cot. Life with two, three or four young children becomes less of a quest for perfection, and more of a juggling act.

So, to summarise:

- There is scientific evidence that babies who are left alone to cry are stressed, and that prolonged crying for weeks and months is harmful.
- Babies are not manipulative. When they are upset, they are upset. They are not 'putting it on' to 'get what they want'.
- You can't teach independence. Children learn that for themselves. Trying too soon makes them clingier.
- Children's need for reassurance doesn't switch off at night.

And:

- Happy parents make for happy children.
- If you don't like something about life, be it your situation, your parenting or your child's behaviour, you are allowed to try and change it.

If you accept these basic principles of childhood development, then you're not going to go far wrong. If you're happier using a cot, use one. And if you've put the time in to give your baby a happy, secure start in life, then who am I to say that you shouldn't try to train your toddler out of waking up at 3 am?

What about those fashionably strict babycare routines?

'Securely attached' children have parents whose attentions are prompt, consistent and appropriate. Now I interpret that to mean prompt to answer a baby's cries, consistently available for the child, day and night, and appropriately able to cuddle, sing or breastfeed a baby to sleep. You won't read that in some other babycare books. They emphasise the importance of promptly following a routine and consistently setting appropriate conditions for solitary sleep.

Routines work by pre-empting a baby's needs, and for some mothers and babies they work very well. The baby never ends up screaming tired and hungry because before he reaches that point, he's already been fed and laid in his cot. Any kind of childcare where mother and baby are both happy is better than one where they aren't.

But if you evaluate routine parenting in the light of Gerhardt's conclusions about infant development, then the practice starts to look more questionable. It's good for a baby to have needs, and to learn to express them, because when you let your baby show you what he wants, it helps him to learn about himself. *This interaction is a vital part of his emotional development.* Sure, some of the job of parenting is about anticipating needs, but that doesn't mean you have to replace them.

Babies thrive on loving cuddles. Eye contact, playing with your face, being on your lap, being involved with everything you do (badly) as you struggle around the house or the shops; these are the ways that babies become social beings. It's not particularly natural for a baby to have to wake up in his cot without being picked up and hugged. It might fit better with the sleep training, but it's another cuddle missed. When eye contact is forbidden during designated nap times, a child gains sleep, but misses out on interaction.

Still, when psychologists bang on about babies with extreme cortisol levels and insecure attachment, they are talking about a major breakdown in the mother-child bond. It is important to be aware that it can happen, but you don't have to let fear affect your confidence. Trust yourself to muddle through and find your own way.

That muddled feeling is what many parents find so difficult. I mean, you love your child. There are a bewildering number of different opinions out there, and almost every new mother feels radically unsure of herself and worries about her choices. You're meant to feel like this. There is an evolutionary advantage in worrying:

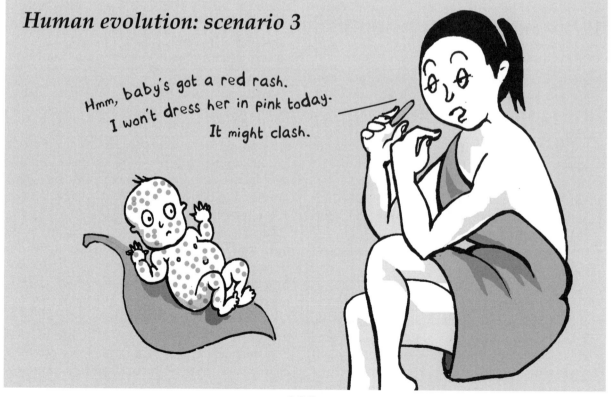

Human evolution: scenario 3

Hmm, baby's got a red rash. I won't dress her in pink today. It might clash.

128

Human evolution: scenario 4

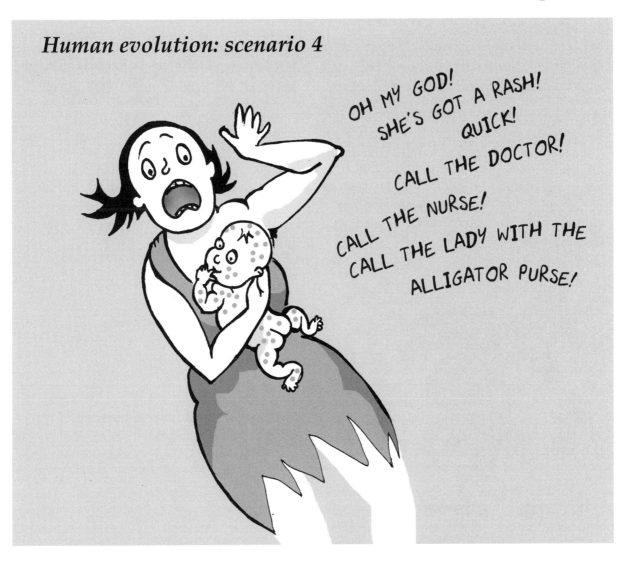

Guess which mother you are descended from?

Continually questioning whether you are doing right by your child is part of what makes you a good parent. Whatever style of parenting you choose, as long as you care about and connect with your baby, that's good enough.

Feeling sensitive?

This is a personal observation, but it seems like a lot of pregnant women and new mothers live in a heightened emotional state, where they are more alert to danger than they ever used to be. Have you ever screamed at your partner to get away from the kerb even though there are blatantly no cars anywhere near? Do you shrink from gory horror films, and turn over to a gardening programme instead? Does the sight of a man carrying a small child on a news report reduce you to tears? There may be an evolutionary reason for all this.

Human beings survive by taking risks. You have to climb trees if you want to gather coconuts, for example. However, we live in social groups. If a pregnant woman or new mother in the tribe were to refuse to climb coconut trees, and instead persuaded other people to take such risks for her, then this exaggerated-risk-perception mother would be less likely to accidentally die than her risk-taking counterparts. So her children would be more likely to survive. And we would be descended from them.

So maybe all our amygdalas go a little bit hyper when we have kids. And they're meant to.

Just a thought.

Oh I can't watch. And to think that I used to climb coconut trees myself.

130

Ouch! Common breastfeeding complaints

"The breasts, especially after delivery, are liable to divers diseases; as

inflammations, excoriations, indurations, tumefactions, nodes, abseses, schirrufes..."

A supplement to Mr Chambers' Cyclopedia, ed. George Lewis Scott 1753

I was hoping that you weren't going to need to read this section. For many women, breastfeeding is a completely pain-free experience. I have to admit though that, among my friends, they're in the minority.

The good news is that none of the complaints listed in this chapter will affect your baby. Breastfeeding is vital to the survival of the species.

The bad news is that they *hurt*, with a particularly unrelenting kind of pain. If you sprain your ankle, then you can rest up for a while until it gets better. But if you crack your nipple, that baby is still going to need feeding every couple of hours... Paracetamol is safe to take when breastfeeding, as long as your baby is healthy and full term. Ibruprofen should be your second choice for pain relief, and you can take it in combination with paracetamol. Don't take aspirin while breastfeeding unless your doctor prescribes it.

But the other good news is that most of the conditions listed here are temporary and curable. By a combination of bad luck and bad advice I had nearly all of these problems, and I still rate my breastfeeding experience as brilliant. In fact, I'm so enthusiastic about it that I had to write a book on the subject. So either I'm a masochistic weirdo, or it is worth persevering (through gritted teeth at times) when breastfeeding goes wrong. Just remember that breastfeeding can be so good when it goes right.

Do you have nipple pain?

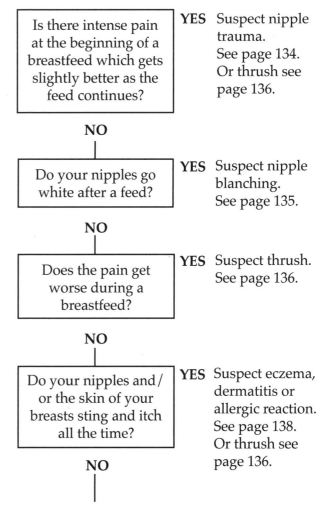

Is there intense pain at the beginning of a breastfeed which gets slightly better as the feed continues? — **YES** Suspect nipple trauma. See page 134. Or thrush see page 136.

NO

Do your nipples go white after a feed? — **YES** Suspect nipple blanching. See page 135.

NO

Does the pain get worse during a breastfeed? — **YES** Suspect thrush. See page 136.

NO

Do your nipples and/or the skin of your breasts sting and itch all the time? — **YES** Suspect eczema, dermatitis or allergic reaction. See page 138. Or thrush see page 136.

NO

Ask a lactation consultant to help.

Do you have breast pain?

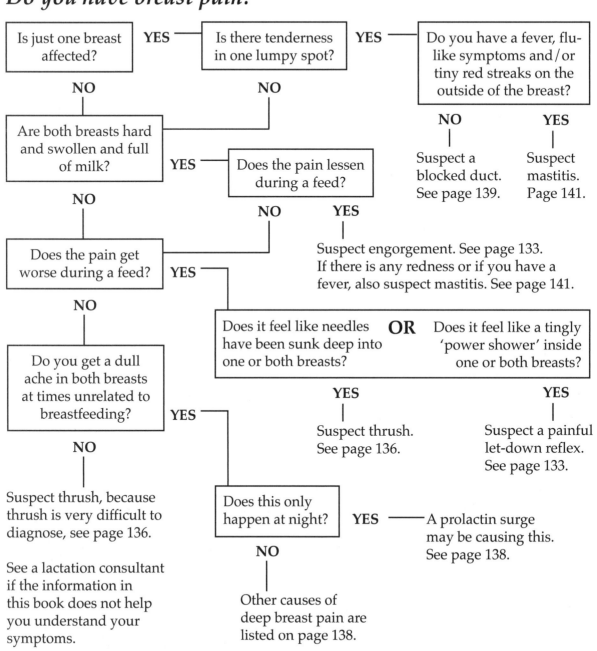

Is just one breast affected? — **YES** — Is there tenderness in one lumpy spot? — **YES** — Do you have a fever, flu-like symptoms and/or tiny red streaks on the outside of the breast?

NO (from "Is just one breast affected?")

NO (from "Is there tenderness in one lumpy spot?")

NO — Suspect a blocked duct. See page 139.

YES — Suspect mastitis. Page 141.

Are both breasts hard and swollen and full of milk? — **YES** — Does the pain lessen during a feed?

NO (from "Are both breasts hard and swollen and full of milk?")

NO (from "Does the pain lessen during a feed?")

YES — Suspect engorgement. See page 133. If there is any redness or if you have a fever, also suspect mastitis. See page 141.

Does the pain get worse during a feed? — **YES**

Does it feel like needles have been sunk deep into one or both breasts? **OR** Does it feel like a tingly 'power shower' inside one or both breasts?

NO (from "Does the pain get worse during a feed?")

YES — Suspect thrush. See page 136.

YES — Suspect a painful let-down reflex. See page 133.

Do you get a dull ache in both breasts at times unrelated to breastfeeding? — **YES**

NO (from "Do you get a dull ache in both breasts at times unrelated to breastfeeding?")

Suspect thrush, because thrush is very difficult to diagnose, see page 136.

See a lactation consultant if the information in this book does not help you understand your symptoms.

Does this only happen at night? — **YES** — A prolactin surge may be causing this. See page 138.

NO — Other causes of deep breast pain are listed on page 138.

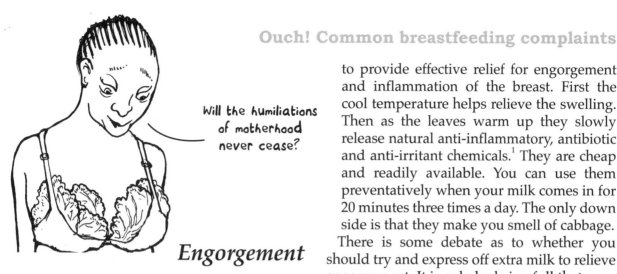

Will the humiliations of motherhood never cease?

Engorgement

This often happens in the first week after the birth. Your breasts get overenthusiastic and produce more milk than your baby can drink. They become painful, round and hard, the skin is taut and shiny and they may feel hot. Your boyfriend thinks they look lovely. You have to resist the urge to slap him.

What to do:

- Ignore the boyfriend.
- Feed the baby as frequently as you can. If she is finding it difficult to latch on, then hand express just enough milk first to soften your nipple.
- Cooling gel packs or bags of frozen peas will help relieve the pain.

And now, it's time for some cabbage leaves down the bra...

- Buy a green cabbage – Savoy is good.
- Rinse the leaves and put them in the fridge.
- When they're cold, take them out, trim the big rib flat with a knife and bash them a bit with a rolling pin or similar.
- Cover your breasts with them, along to the armpits if they're sore too. Hold in place with a supportive bra. Change them every half an hour. Cabbage leaves have been proven to provide effective relief for engorgement and inflammation of the breast. First the cool temperature helps relieve the swelling. Then as the leaves warm up they slowly release natural anti-inflammatory, antibiotic and anti-irritant chemicals.[1] They are cheap and readily available. You can use them preventatively when your milk comes in for 20 minutes three times a day. The only down side is that they make you smell of cabbage.

There is some debate as to whether you should try and express off extra milk to relieve engorgement. It is only by being full that your breasts will get the message to reduce supply, so expressing milk makes the condition last longer. Don't, initially. A warm shower may help the pain, and you can take ibruprofen up to the recommended dose. If engorgement persists for a week or more then discuss the block-feeding strategy on page 77 with your midwife or lactation consultant.

The other time women commonly become engorged is when they wean their child. At this point it is worth remembering that alcohol reduces your milk production. Go on, you've given up breastfeeding, have a drink!

Forceful let down

This is a rare cause of deep breast pain which can also happen in the first weeks when your milk supply is a bit enthusiastic. It feels like a painful 'power shower' tingling inside the breasts when you feed. There isn't very much you can do about this except to wait for everything to calm down, although a couple of glasses of wine a week might help. Try deep breathing relaxation techniques. If you have an overabundant milk supply, see page 77.

133

Nipple trauma

Prevention here is better than cure, so let's have a look at the causes of sore nipples:

- Trying to toughen up your nipples during pregnancy will only cause, not prevent sore nipples. Nipples don't crack because the skin isn't tough enough, they crack because the baby isn't latched on right.
- Blisters on the tip of the nipple. These are caused by the baby's tongue rubbing on the tip of your nipple. Basically, he's not on far enough. These are more common in the early days, especially if the baby has a tongue tie or a short tongue. They may also develop if an older baby gets distracted and tries to feed without latching on properly.
- Blisters on the tip of the nipple and cracks round the side of the nipple. These happen when a baby is very poorly attached, and the mother's nipple moves in and out of his mouth as he suckles. OW! OW! OW!
- Cracks at the side of the nipple. If you get the baby latched on well but then hold her wonkily on the breast, the skin at the junction with the areola can become stressed and crack. This can happen at any time if you feed your baby in a funny position. Say you're feeding your baby lying on your side, then you start watching TV over your shoulder... you end up twisting your body slightly... the breast pulls sideways at your baby's mouth... STOP. Wherever and in whatever position you end up feeding your baby, always make sure that her mouth is square onto your breast.
- Using a hand breast pump too enthusiastically can also crack your nipples. You can hire hospital grade electric pumps, which are gentler, to use until they heal.

What to do:
- *Breathe out* while you latch the baby on. Cracked nipples are sorest at the beginning of a feed, then the pain eases off as the oxytocin kicks in.
- If you are really dreading the next feed then take paracetamol and/or ibruprofen up to the dose recommended on the packet. Don't take aspirin while you are breastfeeding.
- Don't worry if your nipples are bleeding because it shouldn't affect or harm the baby.
- If you are suffering from blisters then improve your latch. Try pushing your nipple upwards with your thumb so baby gets a good mouthful of the underside of your breast. Visit a lactation consultant or a breastfeeding counsellor. Having an experienced woman evaluate what you do will increase your confidence. If you find it easier to latch your baby on well in one position (for example, the Rugby Ball hold) then just use that one for a few days and see if the soreness improves.
- If your nipple has cracked then change the baby's position. Certain positions will be more painful, because the baby's mouth will rub against the crack and reopen it. For example, if the crack occurred when you were lying down (watching telly) then when you feed using that position again it will traumatise the wound. So you will have to sit up and use the Rugby Ball or Cradle hold every single time until the wound has healed. (Damn. No sleep.)
- If you are more comfortable expressing milk from a sore nipple you can choose to do that every three hours and feed off the other breast until it improves.
- When a scab forms on the thin skin of your nipples, it's liable to crack off at the first

134

opportunity and make the wound worse. A good solution is to use a technique called moist wound healing. Get hold of some pure lanolin-based nipple cream. There are several brands available: Lansinoh, Medela PureLan and Medilan. After a feed, wash your hands and smear a thin layer of ointment over the sore place. You don't have to wash this off before you feed the baby, and it's hypoallergenic. The lanolin will prevent a scab from forming and help the cut heal.

- If you can't find any lanolin-based ointment, don't use another sort of nipple cream as it won't work the same way. Instead you can try squeezing some drops of breastmilk onto the crack to help it to heal. Breastmilk has healing and anti-infective properties, so you can use it on any kind of wound. Probably only on someone you know well though.
- You can try nipple shields as an absolute last resort if your nipples are so damaged that you just can't feed any other way. Don't use them for any longer than you have to, as they interfere with your feeding technique and milk supply.
- If the crack just won't heal with moist wound healing or nipple shields and forms a 'crater' then you might have thrush in the wound.
- Air will help the soreness heal. Synthetic bras or soggy nipple pads won't help. You can cut the handles off some plastic tea strainers and put them in your bra to let the air circulate.

No, the humiliations of motherhood will never cease.

Nipple blanching

A baby who isn't latched on properly can squash your nipple and make it go white. This hurts. If this is the case your nipple will be flattened at the end of the feed, and it may have a white stripe across the tip.

- Try to improve the baby's attachment.
- Sometimes babies clamp down on the breast to halt a really strong flow of milk. You can try leaning backwards as described on page 77 if you have this problem.

Some women experience nipple blanching after a feed, or between feeds, or during pregnancy. This is nothing to do with the way your baby feeds – it just happens. The nipples turn white as the blood vessels in the breast constrict, in severe cases they turn blue, then they go red with throbbing or burning pains or numbness. This is often triggered by cold, the same way that your fingers turn white on a cold day.

Vasospasm (to give it its medical name) is more common in women who have already suffered nipple trauma or thrush, who have had breast surgery, or have lupus, rheumatoid arthritis, fibromyalgia or endocrine disease. If you know you already suffer from Raynaud's phenomenon, this is basically the same deal. It can also be caused by smoking, drinking caffeine or taking the Pill.

If this isn't too painful then there's nothing to worry about. If it is, the following suggestions may help:

- Wrap up warm. Cover your breasts quickly after a feed and stick a hot water bottle up your jumper.
- Take ibruprofen if you are really suffering.

135

- Vitamin B6 supplements and evening primrose or fish oil capsules work, but they can take about six weeks to take effect.
- Your doctor can prescribe a low dose of the hypertension drug nifedipine which is safe to use while breastfeeding. Take it for two weeks, then stop for two weeks. Repeat if the symptoms return.[2]

Thrush

Aaaagh! What did your excited friends and relatives buy you to celebrate the new arrival? Sparkling wine? A large box of chocolates? A lovely cake? Did they give any thought to the Candida Albicans fungus that might be lurking in your system, ready to feast on such delights?

We all carry the fungus that causes thrush. Usually it is kept in check by healthy bacteria in our gut. However, antibiotic or steroid drugs, too much sugar, alcohol or the hormonal changes of pregnancy can all make the Candida fungus riot out of control.

Thrush can infect your nipples, your breasts and your baby's mouth and bottom. It can come on at any time, although it is particularly common after antibiotic treatment, which is particularly common after caesarean birth. It can be quite tricky to diagnose correctly, so any time breastfeeding suddenly becomes painful, check for thrush.

Look in your baby's mouth. Little white spots are a giveaway sign. They look like the little curds of milk that she'll usually have in her spit, except that these can't be brushed away with a cotton bud. A mild case of thrush may just show as a whitish bloom on her tongue. A severe case will hurt her and make her cry and pull away when she feeds.

Thrush will also pass into her poo and can cause a bright red, shiny nappy rash, sometimes with blisters or flat orange blotches.

Even if your baby shows no sign of thrush, you can still get thrush on your nipples. They might change colour slightly – if you have dark skin they may go pale pink, and if you have light skin they might go red. They may be shiny or flaky and painful or itchy. (These symptoms are similar to eczema or dermatitis – it can sometimes be difficult to tell.) Or they may hurt, but look no different to normal.

If you have a cracked nipple that refuses to heal, then you could have developed thrush in the wound. I'm sending you some sympathy!

Even if your nipples show no signs of thrush, you can still get thrush in your breast. This feels quite distinctive – like someone has submerged some needles or broken glass deep within it. It can radiate out into your armpit or back. The pain starts in the breast that is being fed from, might get worse during the feed and can continue for some time afterwards. (Forceful let-down pain, which it can be confused with, is more likely to affect both breasts and stops at the end of a feed).

You can repeatedly pass thrush back and forth from you to the baby so both of you have to be treated, regardless of whether you both show symptoms. Thrush varies in severity from a mild condition that will clear up easily, to a horrible painful lingering thing that you need to blitz with nuclear-strength chemicals and severe lifestyle changes, so the remedies here are arranged in order from simple things to try first, all the way up to serious measures for the desperate. If you have severe breast pain, skip to the end.

- Eat some natural, live yoghurt – the acidophilus good bacteria are active against thrush. You can put this on your nipples too, after a feed.
- If you or your baby are prescribed antibiotics or steroids it is a good idea to get an acidophilus supplement from a healthfood shop to restore gut flora to health.
- Don't express breastmilk onto a sore nipple as you would if it was cracked – thrush loves breastmilk.
- Change soggy breast pads often as thrush loves moist warmth. Let your nipples air.
- Wash your hands well before you feed the baby, and again after you change his nappy.
- Leave his nappy off for a few hours if his bottom is sore. You can safely put yoghurt on his bottom too.
- Don't use any soaps, baby lotions, baby bath, baby shampoo or baby wipes for a while. Wash him in plain water, or water with a splash of cider vinegar in.
- Nappy creams that contain tea tree or calendula are both active against thrush so you can use these on his bottom.
- Boil some water for 20 minutes, so it's sterile, then add one teaspoon of bicarbonate of soda to one cup of water. Swab this around your baby's mouth and over your nipples with a piece of clean cotton wool. Repeat this for a few days until you see an improvement.
- Grapefruit seed extract is a natural antifungal substance. Again boil some water for 20 minutes, then dilute the extract as directed on the packet for use as a mouthwash. Swab your baby's mouth and your nipples repeatedly.
- Don't drink any alcohol at all – thrush loves alcohol.

Any improvement? Yes? No? Right, more hardcore solutions:

- The thrush fungus can survive outside your body on your clothes so you need to wash your bras, any washable breast pads, milky t-shirts and nappies on the hottest setting you can. Ironing also kills it. I'll let you off washing and ironing the nappies if you're using disposables.
- You can take paracetamol and ibruprofen, together if you need to, for the pain.
- Dummies harbour thrush so stop using them, or buy extra, change them frequently, and boil them for 20 minutes after use.
- If you have vaginal thrush then treat yourself and your partner, regardless of whether they show symptoms.
- See your doctor for a prescription for antifungal gel for your nipples and your baby's mouth. This will work for sore nipples, but may or may not be effective for thrush that is actually inside your breast.
- The thrush in your system is affected by the food that you eat. It would make sense to lay off the yeast extract or nutritional yeast flakes.
- Gentian violet is a traditional remedy that is extremely effective against thrush. Use a 1% solution, or weaker, and paint it over your nipples and inside baby's mouth with a clean paintbrush or cotton bud. It is messy and stains clothes and skin purple. Reapply a further time once the stain has faded, by which time there should be a marked improvement. It is difficult to buy gentian violet in this country because very large doses cause cancer in rats; however, it has a proven track record as a safe remedy for thrush in babies.[3] Best saved for occasional use.

Is this working yet? Brilliant! No? Oh, OK:

- Sorry, I hate to say this, but Candida Albicans feeds on sugar and bread (which contains yeast). Women with thrush commonly crave bread and sweet things, which is actually the evil yeast inside them demanding to be fed! If you suffer badly from recurrent thrush then it may be worth making some pretty radical changes to your diet. Start with cutting down on sugary foods, fruit juices and bread and see if it makes an improvement.
- Your doctor can prescribe a systemic anti-fungal treatment to be taken internally by you and your partner. This is usually only necessary if you have thrush inside your breasts, where anti-fungal gels and creams can't reach. The most effective drug is fluconazole.

  Unfortunately fluconazole is not licensed for use by breastfeeding mothers because it passes into your breastmilk. Duh! That's the whole point! It has to pass into your breastmilk – that's why it's so effective. The anti-fungal agent in your milk then goes on to treat the baby at the same time. The drug is licensed to be directly given to babies in doses ten times higher than the traces in your milk.[4] The World Health Organisation recognises that it is safe for use when breastfeeding, but the UK drugs safety bodies don't.[5,6]

  This just makes me so cross. Here is a serious condition that is adversely affecting thousands of mothers and babies and two of the most effective treatments – gentian violet and fluconazole – are not readily available to the women who need them.

  Your doctor may still prescribe fluconazole 'off-label' if you need it. Show her the references on page 200. Fluconazole works.
- Throw away any milk that you have expressed and frozen while you had thrush in case it reinfects you both.

Other causes of nipple pain

Eczema or dermatitis may also cause itchy, flaky painful nipples. This is usually a reaction to something you have put on your nipples. If you have recently started using a nipple cream or ointment, then stop. Change your washing powder. Don't use soap or perfume on your breasts. Avoid plastic-backed breast pads. Eczema can also be triggered by eating foods that you are allergic to. Hydrocortisone cream is available on prescription as a last resort.

Other causes of breast pain

If you don't have any tender lumps in your breasts, and are experiencing pain at various times, consider these causes and solutions:

- Women with very large breasts may find that their breasts and back ache when breastfeeding. A well-fitting and no doubt extremely expensive bra can help – some women find it helps to wear one at night too. Supporting your breasts from underneath with a fitted top or waistcoat around your abdomen could relieve the pressure on your upper back. Yoga classes can ease back pain. You can take paracetamol and ibruprofen.
- It is quite common to feel a deep ache in your breasts at night. This is a surge of prolactin hormone ramping up your milk supply and nothing to worry about.
- An old injury or surgery can cause lactating breasts to ache. Massage may help.

Blocked ducts

Your milk lobes form in clusters inside your breast, each one with a tube, or duct, which runs out of the end of your nipple. When one of these ducts become blocked, the lobes behind it swell up painfully with trapped milk.

Pain from a blocked duct comes on suddenly. You sit down and undo your bra, and you feel a twinge in one of your breasts. On closer inspection there is a hard, lumpy painful mass in there. Don't freak out. This is quite common. As long as you don't have a fever or flu-like symptoms, treating a blocked duct is quite straightforward.

What has happened is that one or more of your milk ducts have been squashed shut for a little while, and the milk in there has formed a little plug of cream cheese. The milk ducts have filled up with milk that has nowhere to go. This could get better by itself, but if it doesn't then you'll get mastitis.

Blocked ducts are often caused by pressure on the breast, say by:

- Pressing your fingers into your breast while breastfeeding.
- Squashing your breast into an unusual position.
- Wearing a bra that is too small, or one with underwire in that cuts into the milk lobes.
- Sleeping on your front.

- The straps from a baby carrier.
- Pressure from a seat belt.

This list could go on and on. You generally won't notice what it was that caused the blockage until it has already happened.

It seemed to me that I tended to get blocked ducts when I was rushing around doing too much. Of course, I can't back this up with a scientific analysis of the physiology of milk blockage – it's just a personal observation. Take a blocked duct as a sign that you need to take it easy and take care of yourself.

What to do:

- Well, babies are generally quite good at getting milk out of a breast, although this may be part of the problem. If your attachment and positioning are poor then the baby will have trouble draining all the lobes of the breast efficiently. If this is the case then sore nipples and frequent feeds are likely to be a problem as well as blocked ducts. Make an appointment with a breastfeeding specialist.
- For the same reason, you are more likely to get blocked ducts in your baby's least favourite breast – see page 144 for tips to deal with this.
- Because the baby milks the breast with his tongue, the area under his chin is drained most efficiently at each feed. So, the next time he is hungry put him straight onto the breast with the blockage, with his chin pointing to the lumpy bit. This could mean lying down and positioning the baby upside down! Leaning-forward positions may also help your milk flow faster. There are pictures on page 151.

- If you can't position the baby like this for some reason – let's say you happen to be on a crowded train – then feed the baby in whatever position you find easiest, and use your free hand to gently massage the blockage from the outside in towards the nipple.
- If the lump is on the underside of your breast then loosen your bra completely and put a rolled up cloth nappy or tea towel under your breast while you feed. This helps the lobes drain.

If at the end of the feed the tender lump has dissipated, then the problem is solved. If not, then it's time to take more action:

- Apply warmth to the breast. You can get in a hot bath or shower, or apply a compress to the breast. A 21st century way of making a hot compress is to pour some hot water onto a disposable nappy and then lay the wet side over the sore place. Have it as hot as you can bear without burning yourself.
- Have a look at your nipple. Is there a tiny white spot on the end of it? That means that the blockage has moved down to the end of the duct and is ready to burst. Try soaking it in warm water, then briskly rubbing it with a clean dry flannel. Once it pops, the release of the pressure may cause a jet of milk to shoot out across the room, so have a towel handy.
- Other ways of dislodging the spot include scraping it or popping it with a sterilized needle, but be careful not to damage your nipple.
- If there is nothing unusual on your nipple, then the blockage is deeper inside your breast.

You can use massage to encourage it to move along the duct. Place two or three fingers flat on your breast. Start on the outside of the blockage and massage in towards the nipple making small circular movements. Don't let your fingers slide over the skin. The idea is to be firm enough to apply some pressure but not so rough that you bruise yourself. You can combine this with gentle use of a breast pump if you have one. Keep checking your nipple to see if you can see the blockage yet.

- If your blocked duct is very painful, ibruprofen will help the pain and inflammation.

Massage, warmth and pumping should be enough to make a difference. If you try this and don't see any results, then wait until the baby is hungry again. Feed off the sore breast first again, then swap to the other side if that breast is becoming uncomfortable too. Repeat the heat and massage. As the pressure builds up in the lobes, the blockage should become easier to shift.

Usually once the little white spot pops then all the lobes will drain, sometimes quite spectacularly. Gently massage that quarter of the breast with your whole hand and check that all the lumpiness has gone. Sometimes there are a series of blockages in the same duct and you need to repeat the heat and massage until they have all cleared. You can even end up with creamy spaghetti stuff coming out of that duct. Freaky, huh?

Recurrent blocked ducts might be helped by drinking a dash of cider vinegar in a pint of water every day. This old wives' remedy won't do you any harm.

'A severe gathered bosom is always ushered in with a shivering fit… either accompanied or followed by sharp lancinating pains of the bosom. The breast now greatly enlarges, becomes hot and is very painful.'

Advice to Wife and Mother

Mastitis

Should you at any time suddenly feel very unwell, with flu-like aching, a fever and a tender lumpy mass in one breast, then you have mastitis. Tiny red streaks may appear on the sore part of the breast. Go to bed with the baby and take paracetamol, ibruprofen or both for the sharp, lancinating pains.

Mastitis can be caused by an infection or a blockage. The symptoms are exactly the same. A cracked nipple, for example, could allow an infection to travel into the milk lobes – if you see any sign of infection on your nipples then see a doctor or lactation consultant without delay. Alternatively, if a blocked duct refuses to shift, then milk will start to spill out of the overfill lobes into your bloodstream. Annoyingly, your body reacts to the milk protein as if it were foreign invading germs: it sends plenty of white blood cells over to inflame the area and gives you a fever to kill off the germs.

You have various treatment options here and you might need all of them:

- Feed the baby from the infected side first every time, swapping to the other breast enough to keep that one comfortable too. Use a breast pump between feeds. You may notice that the milk you express has a greenish layer, if so, discard it.
- The inflammation may make your milk salty. This won't harm the baby, but he might not like the taste. If he refuses the breast, then enrol your partner to help drain the breast. This is an emergency here.
- Keep up the hot compresses and massage but be very gentle. Don't let your fingers slide over the skin. You can combine this with hand expression or gentle pumping.
- If your breast is reddened try the homeopathic remedy Belladonna. If it is pale, try Bryonia.
- Get the cabbage leaves out again (see page 133). Use them cold from the fridge, or blanch briefly in boiling water or run a hot iron over them. Hey, back when you were pregnant, I bet you never imagined you'd be ironing cabbage leaves before the year was out!
- Drink plenty of water and keep taking the painkillers.
- If your symptoms do not improve within 24 hours then see a doctor without delay. Your GP can prescribe you antibiotics, which are usually effective for mastitis. It's common to be told, even by a doctor, to stop breastfeeding from the affected side, but this is the worst thing to do. Try to get as much milk out of the breast as possible, or an abscess could develop.
- Antibiotics work by reducing the infection and the inflammation (ibruprofen helps for this too). However, there are some instances where they don't help. This is because the underlying blockage just keeps pumping milk out into the bloodstream. In this case try a session of acupuncture by someone trained in Traditional

Chinese Medicine. I don't know why this works, but then I haven't been developing a holistic system of medicine for more than two thousand years. Acupuncture needles are very fine – it's nothing like having an injection. You'll need a friend to go with you to mind the baby. At the very least acupuncture will make you feel calm and relaxed.

- As with blocked ducts, recurrent mastitis may be linked to poor feeding technique. Your baby may not be draining the breast efficiently. Seek professional help.
- Take a probiotic such as acidophilus or live yoghurt after you complete the course of antibiotics to reduce the risk of thrush.
- If an injury or surgical scar seems to be causing recurrent blocked ducts or mastitis in one particular place, try ultrasound therapy.

Abscess

If you don't receive effective treatment for mastitis then an abscess can develop. This is a pocket of pus which forms around the affected lobes. It's not very common. It is very painful.

You may need to take prescription painkillers and if you do, you and your baby will be slightly drowsy, so make sure that she feeds regularly, and put her in a cot to sleep. If taking an opiate-based painkiller makes you feel very strange or makes your baby extremely sleepy then contact your doctor without delay. Adverse reactions to codeine and opiates may require the administration of an antidote.

If the abscess is very close to your nipple it may temporarily be too painful for you to feed from that side. If you can file a section out of the flange of a breast pump, you may still be able to express milk.

Surgical drainage is the recommended treatment. An ultrasound scan may be used to locate the abscess: drain the breast of milk just beforehand to make the scan easier to read.

Breast surgeons tend to want to perform surgery radially around the edge of the nipple area, because the scar is less noticeable. This is rubbish for breastfeeding, as it cuts the milk ducts and nerves, so make sure the incision is lateral, ie in a line pointing away from the nipple. The wound will be packed and dressed after surgery.

While you are waiting for surgery it is possible that the abscess will spontaneously rupture. The pus-filled area gradually works its way to the surface and your skin will go red and shiny and start to peel. Keep applying hot cabbage leaves. At some point, you might find milk dripping out of your breast somewhere other than the nipple. Sorry, this is getting really medieval here!

What I did in this case (I told you I had all of these conditions!) was boil some water for 20 minutes, waited for it to cool slightly and added copious amounts of salt to it. Then I soaked the affected area in bowls of hot salt water until everything had drained out, and successfully avoided an operation.

Once the abscess has healed, those milk lobes will be scarred, so this does affect your milk production ever so slightly. Feed from that side lots, and express milk to build up your supply.

Other lumps

It is possible to develop a tumour in your breast while you are breastfeeding, just as it is at any other time in your life. Examine your breasts regularly, so you are familiar with what is normal for you. Check armpits as well as breasts. 90% of lumps that develop in women's breasts are not cancerous, but they all need to be examined by a medical professional to make sure.

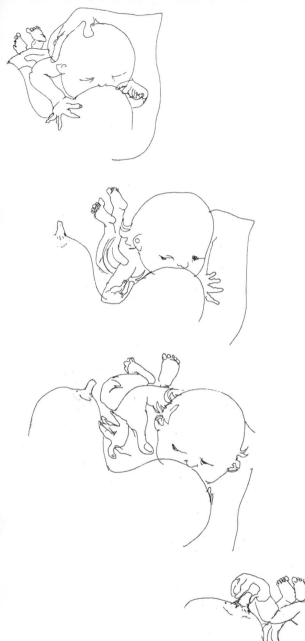

Bad habits

Nipple twiddling

Aaagh! Well before babies find out that all adults carry around with them twinkling musical toys that speak and have buttons to dribble into on the front (mobile phones) they discover another fun toy to play with. Your other nipple. It's always there, it's nice to hold and since nipple stimulation increases milk flow, it helps them get more milk. They have in effect found the volume button.

This used to drive me nuts! There are limits to how much I can do the hippy earth-mother thing. Strangely, my sister-in-law, who is far more conventional than I am, thinks it's funny and cute.

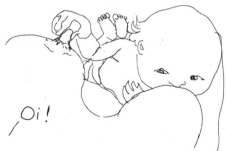

Oi!

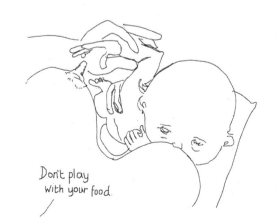

Don't play with your food.

What else? I thought it was cute and funny when my baby started wiggling his feet in bed. Then the wriggling turned into rhythmical kicking. You know how, if you get hit only very lightly but repeatedly in the same place it can get very sore? This sore patch travelled right down my abdomen and thighs as the baby grew. Eventually the glorious day dawned when he was finally long enough for me to pin his legs down with my knee while I was feeding him. Before then I had resorted to tying the feet of his babygro together, or piling pillows over his legs.

Oh, and isn't this one just delightful? Baby is hungry. Baby starts to feed. Something interesting happens, and baby rolls away to have a quick look. Mother, mindful that she is sitting in a crowded restaurant with her nipples on display, pulls her top down. Baby turns back. Baby's favourite nipple has disappeared. Baby is cross. Mother is none too impressed either.

Favouritism

Your baby will probably really love your breasts, but he might not love them equally. Your breasts won't be exactly the same. One may have a faster milk let-down or a differently shaped nipple, and once your baby has decided that that one is HIS FAVOURITE breast, it's quite a job to get him to take the other one.

This happened to me after I got the breast abscess. Baby went right off that breast, only ever wanted the other one, and I needed to use some subterfuge to get him to feed from it again.
- Try to feed baby off the 'unfavourite' breast.
- Give up. Hold him in the Cradle hold and latch him onto the one he likes.
- Wait about a minute, then, quick, swing him round so he's feeding off the other one in the Rugby Ball hold. If you time it right, he'll be so tranced out from the first breast that he'll carry right on with the second one. If you've switched too soon, he'll notice and protest. If you leave it too late, he'll fall asleep the moment you take him off. Damn.

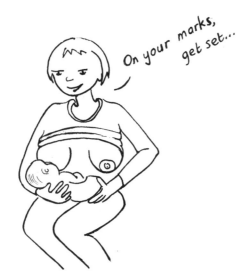

On your marks, get set...

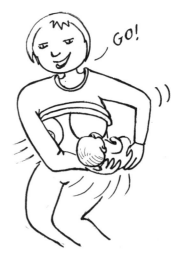

GO!

Biting

There's a strange new edge to feeding a baby after his teeth have come through – a dancing-with-danger kind of thrill. I discovered that babies are mostly very good at not biting their mothers – it must be a survival thing. However, with a strange inevitability, the day did come where I got bit.

Now the books say that you must not, at this point, yell loudly and fling the baby down in case you make him scared to feed. The razor shark bite made me forget anything I ever read in any book. I yelled. I flung. I stormed out of the room. Fortunately he wasn't scared. I do a fair amount of yelling and flinging in my day-to-day childcare (in a nice way!) so maybe he had been inoculated against this kind of extreme reaction. He never bit me again.

That was a tricky situation, and I think I've demonstrated that I handled it very badly. Whether biting goes on to become a repeat problem seems to depend very much on the baby. My little sister, faced with an overwhelming, teething urge to chew, succumbed on quite a few occasions, and I remember my mum dabbing disconsolately at her nipple and commenting that the milk seemed to be coming out of a new hole. A friend had a baby who started to nip her any time he wasn't really hungry, in a crotchety kind of way. She weaned.

Biting doesn't mean that you have to stop breastfeeding though, if you don't want to, as you can teach a baby not to bite.

- This seems a bit counter-intuitive but a good strategy is to pull the baby right *into* the breast when he bites you. Your breast will cover his nose so he can't breathe and he'll open his mouth and let go. Another way to extricate your nipple without further damage is to slip your finger between his jaws.
- Stop the feed. Babies like breastfeeding – they'll soon learn not to do things that end the feed.
- If he's broken the skin (the little varmint!) use the moist wound healing method on page 135.
- Test your teething baby by offering him a finger or a toy to chomp on before trying to feed him. Teething babies can respond well to the homeopathic remedy *Chamomilla*.
- Babies can't bite when they're latched on and feeding well because their tongue will cover their lower teeth. So, they have to lose the latch slightly in order to bite. This subtle movement means that you can spot when Jaws there is about to strike. So pay attention to a cheeky, bitey baby while he feeds. If you suspect that he's getting bored, take him off and play with him for a while, then continue the feed. Give him heaps of praise every time he doesn't bite.
- It is a good idea to say 'No' firmly rather than yell loudly – either your baby might get scared, or he might think it's funny and try biting you again to see the reaction. Good luck with remembering that advice in the heat of the moment.

Out and about

You and your baby are, for the time being, an inseparable biological and social unit. Your baby has a right to eat. You have a right to freedom of movement. Breastfeeding is widely acknowledged to be the best form of nutrition for a baby. You can feed your baby anywhere you want to.

But would you actually want to feed your baby in public? Some women have decidedly mixed feelings about this when they consider it ahead of time.

That will almost certainly change once the baby is here. Breastfeeding is a journey. Initially you may find yourself clutching your baby helplessly thinking 'Oh, no, that's Uncle Colin – I can't possibly breastfeed in front of Uncle Colin!' A few months later you'll be gaily whipping up your t-shirt, popping the baby on and saying 'What? They're just milk production glands, aren't they?' to startled male friends.

I had a relaxed upbringing where my family was comfortable with nudity, but this didn't just happen to me. My sister-in-law Tracey wasn't breastfed, never saw her parents naked as a child, and thinks my family is very strange for having no lock on the bathroom door. Before her baby was born she confided in me:

'I could never breastfeed in front of Adam [her father-in-law]. I'll just have to go and hide upstairs once the baby is born.'

Two months later, at baby Lily's christening, she quite happily put her to the breast in a crowded room.

'Hey Trace, I thought you weren't going to breastfeed in front of anyone else?'

'Yeah, but you know, I'm not really bothered by that now.'

Breastfeeding for the first time in front of male family members is actually more difficult than breastfeeding in public. What does it matter if a stranger catches a brief glimpse of your breast? Undoing your bra in front of your husband's father is infinitely more embarrassing. Especially if he feels the need to break the ice with a few, ill-judged boob jokes.

You've probably seen very few women breastfeeding in public. Do you know why? It's because it isn't very noticeable. Once you've got the hang of latching your baby on quickly you can breastfeed anywhere, and very few people will even know what you are doing. And the only way more women are going to get the confidence to breastfeed in public is if more women do it. Fifty years ago miniskirts were unacceptable. Society can change.

Meeting another breastfeeding mother at a nice cafe is a good way to increase your confidence. If you like, you can practise in front of the mirror before you go out. T-shirts are brilliant for subtle breastfeeding – they are soft, easy to lift and they drape well over your breasts. Shirts that open at the front are less useful but you can try leaving the top few buttons done up. With some clothes you have to take your breast out over the neckline, but once the baby is latched on, you're not exposing any more of yourself than you would in a low-cut top. Accessorise with a scarf, shawl or cardigan if you want. Vest type tops with large arm holes are good – you can pass the baby in through the side. Try draping a muslin over your shoulder for concealment. A good sling is a great option.

You can buy purpose-made wraps to cover up with, but they make the mechanics of breastfeeding more complicated. And unless you always feed your baby under a blanket, even at home, then she may not take kindly to being shrouded in cloth. It's good for her to be able to breathe, as well as feed.

Breastfeeding does occasionally mean that you flash a tiny bit of flesh. This is fine. No-one's looking – we're all far too polite for that. Maybe you might catch a little child staring, but that's good, they're seeing something that they need to see. Every time a woman breastfeeds outside the home, the world learns a little more about this wonderful, natural act.

What if someone is offended by you breastfeeding? Well, hey, for any uptight busybody who is prepared to complain about your baby getting nourishment there are loads of people, like me, who think that a baby breastfeeding is amongst the most beautiful sights in the world. You might be surprised by the support you receive.

Me, buying a bacon sandwich in crowded farmer's market while baby screams:
'He'll have to wait. I can't feed him here.'
Old farmer standing next to me in the queue:
'Why not? S'only natural after all.'
(I suppose, on reflection, he'd had plenty of experience of milk production).

Really, worrying that people might disapprove of your breastfeeding is going to mess with your head. When the time comes to feed in a particularly full-on situation – on a crowded bus, for example – don't assume that everyone hates what you are doing. The people around you will avert their eyes. They do this out of respect for your modesty, *not* because they disapprove. If the choice is that your baby screams for forty minutes in the rush hour, or that he receives some comfort at your breast, then you can be sure that you have the 100% backing of those commuters. They'd all rather your child was fed.

It is however, theoretically possible that someone might at some time complain to you about some aspect of your breastfeeding, by asking you to move, to hide, or not to do it at all. Such requests tend to be made by employees of establishments on behalf of some mythical third party who 'might be upset' by you and your baby, without any respect at all for how upsetting this actually is for you, the recipient of such ignorant prejudice. You're a new mother – you deserve society's unquestioned support for doing something that can be so difficult. Your breastfeeding relationship is intensely personal. No-one has a right to comment on it. Ever.

If you are unlucky enough to have this happen to you, keep calm and get a pen and paper. Ask the name of the person giving you attitude, and write that down together with exactly what they have said and the name of the establishment. You'll probably want to leave at that point, and I don't blame you.

Back home, get in touch with the National Childbirth Trust, the La Leche League or another breastfeeding support organisation, and describe your experience. They will endeavour to get you an apology from the member of staff that humiliated you, and a change of company policy to prevent it happening again.

This is a civil rights issue. It is not illegal to feed your baby anywhere they are hungry, and it is discriminatory for someone to stop you. Scotland recently strengthened this by passing a law which makes it illegal for someone to attempt to prevent a woman from breastfeeding. We need more laws like this, protecting the rights of the most vulnerable members of society. They need their milk. Anyhow, anytime and anywhere.

The Mama Sutra –
advanced breastfeeding positions

These are drawn from life. Breastfeeding women can do all this and more!

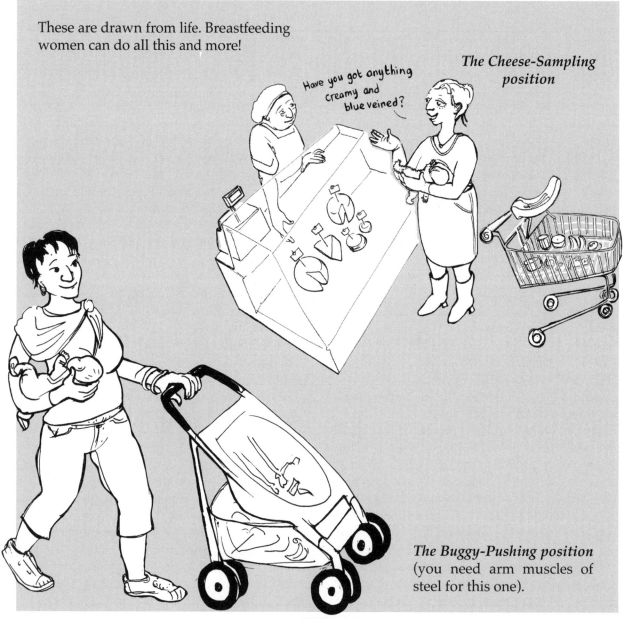

The Cheese-Sampling position

The Buggy-Pushing position (you need arm muscles of steel for this one).

The Addressing-Letters-in-the-Post-Office position

Special Delivery?
No, not really.
Nine hour labour
No complications

nappy
nappy
nappy
nappy
nappy
nappy

The Just-Quickly-Checking-my-emails-in-the-Internet-Cafe position

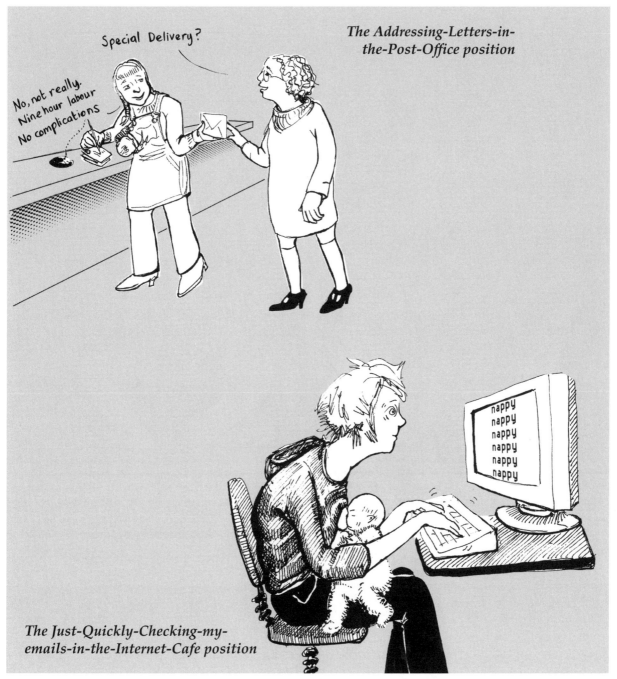

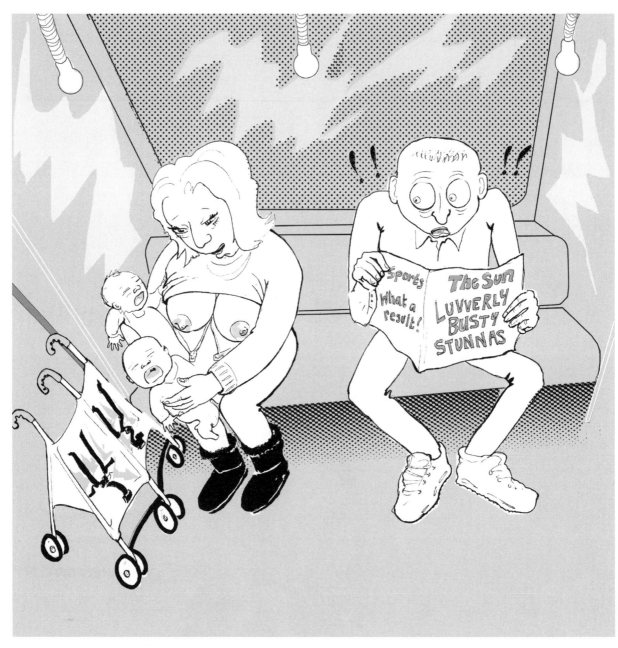

You can't be shy when you're tandem-feeding twins.

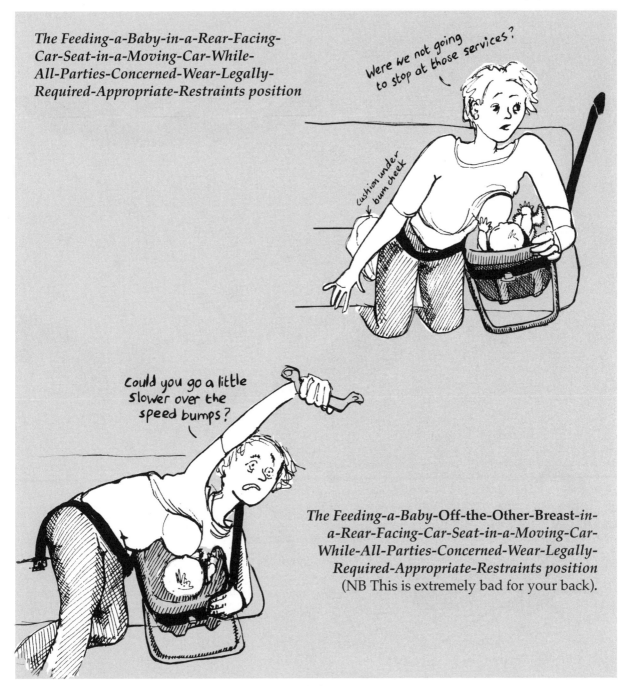

The Feeding-a-Baby-in-a-Rear-Facing-Car-Seat-in-a-Moving-Car-While-All-Parties-Concerned-Wear-Legally-Required-Appropriate-Restraints position

Were we not going to stop at those services?

cushion under bum cheek

Could you go a little slower over the speed bumps?

The Feeding-a-Baby-Off-the-Other-Breast-in-a-Rear-Facing-Car-Seat-in-a-Moving-Car-While-All-Parties-Concerned-Wear-Legally-Required-Appropriate-Restraints position
(NB This is extremely bad for your back).

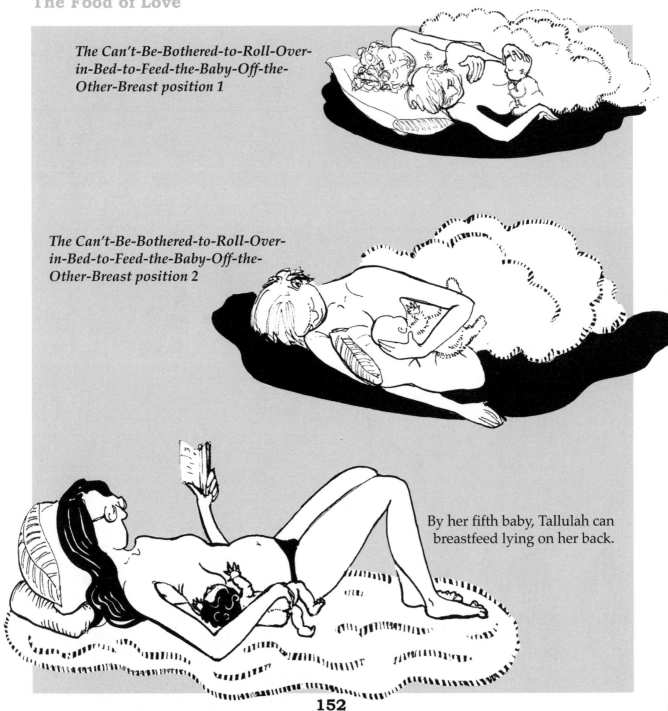

The Can't-Be-Bothered-to-Roll-Over-in-Bed-to-Feed-the-Baby-Off-the-Other-Breast position 1

The Can't-Be-Bothered-to-Roll-Over-in-Bed-to-Feed-the-Baby-Off-the-Other-Breast position 2

By her fifth baby, Tallulah can breastfeed lying on her back.

Some Crazy-Things-you-do-to-Sort-Out-a-Blocked-Duct positions

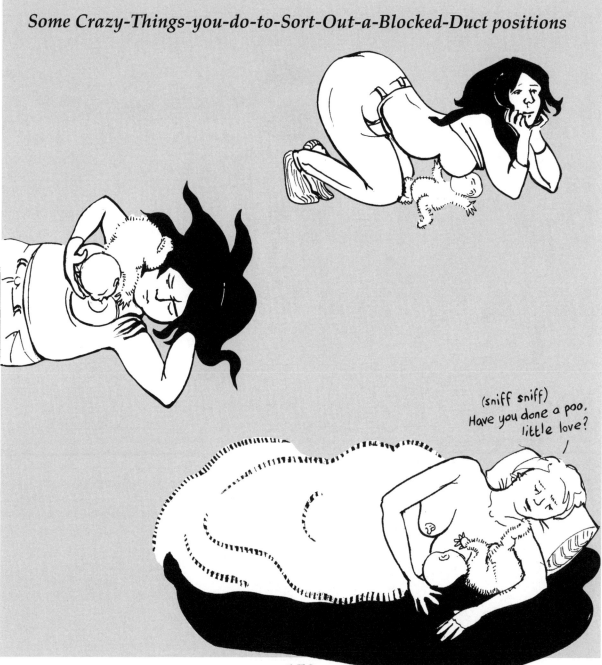

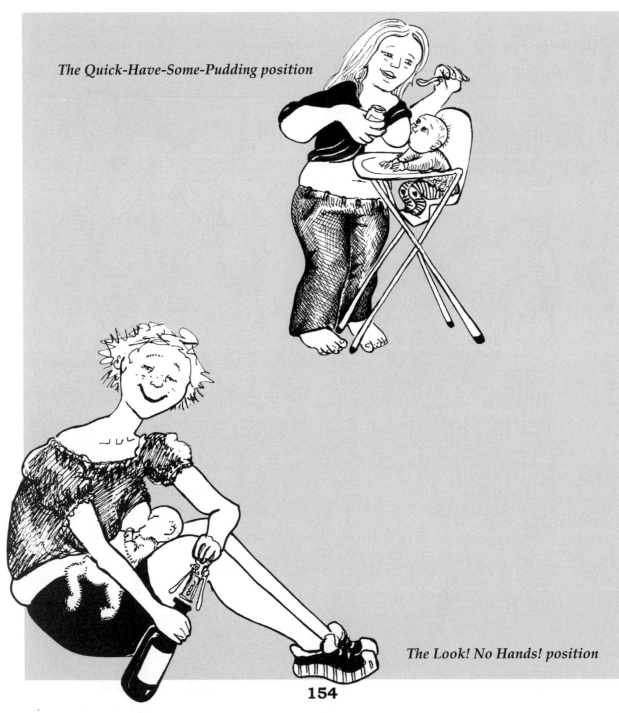

The Quick-Have-Some-Pudding position

The Look! No Hands! position

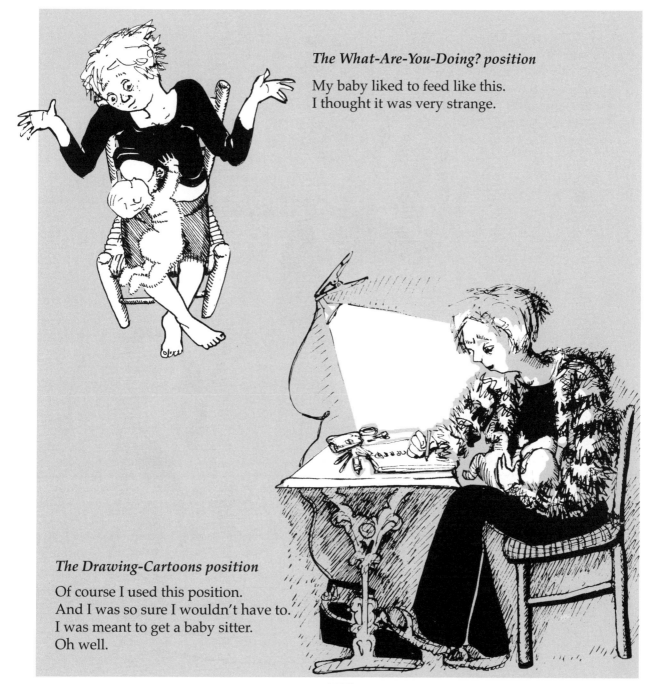

The What-Are-You-Doing? position

My baby liked to feed like this.
I thought it was very strange.

The Drawing-Cartoons position

Of course I used this position.
And I was so sure I wouldn't have to.
I was meant to get a baby sitter.
Oh well.

Make the most of it.
Ring the changes.
Because it won't be long
before you're not positioning
the baby any more –
he's positioning you.

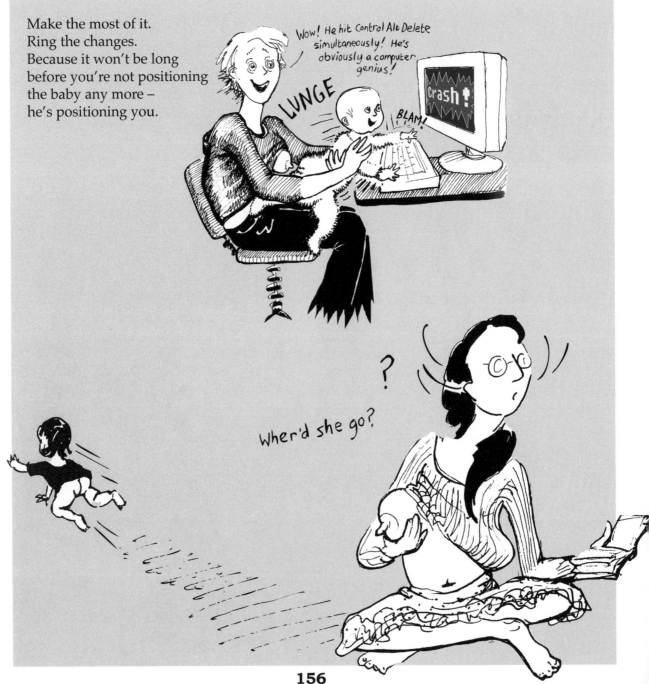

It's a sling thing!

Take an eight-pound (3.6 kg) baby. Strap her into a nine-pound (4 kg) car seat. Clip that to a 25 pound (11 kg) pushchair. You have increased the weight of your baby to three stone, nearly 20 kilos. Now try to walk up a flight of stairs.

Pushchairs are expensive, difficult to clean and are held together with little plastic clips that break after a couple of years, usually at a very awkward moment.

Baby slings are cheap, they go in the washing machine, and provided that you tie the baby in properly, there's no chance that they'll suddenly disintegrate on you in the middle of a shopping trip.

Baby slings also collapse down smaller than pushchairs, and you don't have to fold them to get them on the bus.

Carrying your baby in a car seat, out at arm's length or jammed awkwardly on your hip will make her seem very heavy. Get a sling that ties her in close to your tummy and hips and you'll hardly notice her weight. You've just spent nine months building up the muscles needed to heft a baby around with you. Your new baby is lighter than what you're used to carrying, because you no longer have to lug a placenta and a load of amniotic fluid around too.

Every day your baby will get a little heavier. And, each day, your muscles will become stronger. This is a brilliant thing about carrying babies – the more often you do it, the lighter they're going to feel. When she gets really porky, she'll develop enough upper body strength to be carried in a back pack which will make her seem lighter again.

A newborn baby in a pushchair is alone, in a little plastic-walled bubble. She can't see you. She can't smell you. She can't hear you very clearly. She's down there at the level of the car exhaust fumes, and for you to see to cross the road, you'll have to push her right up close to the traffic. Being strapped into a pushchair with the raincover down is training for spending life isolated in a car. The world speeds by. You can see it, but you can't feel it, or touch it – you can't interact with it.

But when you carry your baby snuggled on your chest she can hear the familiar sound of your heartbeat and feel the movements that comforted her in the womb. Your body heat will warm her. She can hear your voice, and see your lips move, which is excellent training for learning to talk. She can see you. She can see what you're doing. She's part of what you're doing. She can smell you. You smell nice and milky. She can have a little feed. No-one can see.

Sling Girl can leap country stiles, march over hill tops, even navigate the London Underground with ease!

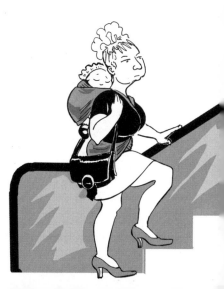

A sling is just a piece of cloth. You can buy specially made ones with buckles and clips, or you can try this very simple wrap, which is cheap, versatile and gives good hip support.

Go out and buy five metres of 100% cotton jersey (t-shirt material) – the sort of fabric that curls up at the edges when you stretch it. Don't buy something with Lycra in, as it doesn't want to be too stretchy. Cut a piece off lengthways, half a metre wide. You'll have enough fabric left over for lots of baby blankets or another sling for a friend.

Now transform yourself into SLING GIRL! These instructions look complicated, but if you can master folding a double stroller or get a seat belt round a car seat correctly, then with practice you can do this too. And don't stop there, www.wearyourbaby.org can show you six more ways of wearing this wrap, including back and hip carries that are great for toddlers.

Breastfeeding a newborn baby on the move

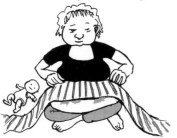

1) Sit cross-legged with a pillow on your lap and a sleepy baby next to you. Find the centre of the cloth and lay it on the pillow.

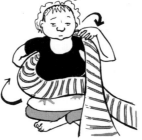

2) Take one end behind your waist and up over the opposite shoulder. Don't twist the cloth. Repeat with the other end.

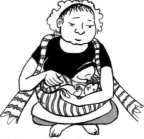

3) Put the baby on your lap and make a little pocket round her with the fabric. Lean forward and latch her on.

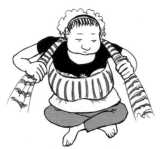

4) Pull the cloth over your shoulders to snuggle the baby in tight. You can trap the ends under your knees or feet to keep the tension.

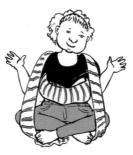

5) Lose the pillow. Sit up. Is the baby well-supported? If so, bring the ends down and cross them over the baby.

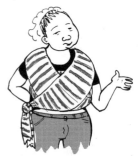

6) Wrap the ends around your waist. Tie them at the back, or at the side, or around at the front if you have a lot of spare cloth.

Breastfeeding a bigger baby on the move

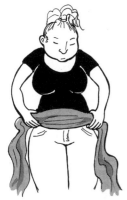

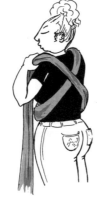

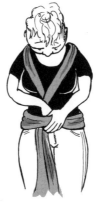

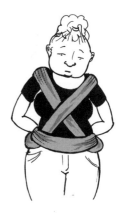

1) Find the centre of the cloth and lay it over your belly button.

2) Take the ends around your waist, cross them over and throw them over your shoulders.

3) Pull the waist-band out and feed the ends through.

4) Make an X on your front and take the ends round your waist again. Either tie them there, on your back or...

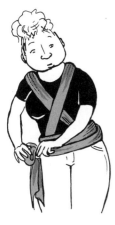

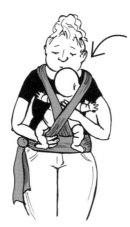

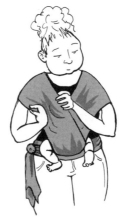

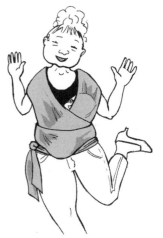

5) ...bring them round to the front and tie them at the side, if you have enough cloth.

6) Feed the baby in through the top of the X and pull the cloth out wide to support her bottom.

7) Stretch out the fabric over your shoulders. If you want you can bring the inner waist-band up over her legs and bottom to make it more snug.

8) Latch her on, and off you go!

Your baby can stay quiet in a sling while you go about your daily tasks. Damn. There goes my excuse for not doing the laundry.

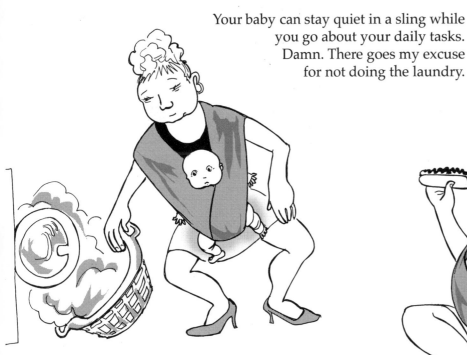

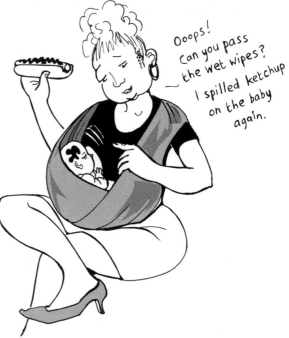

Ooops! Can you pass the wet wipes? I spilled ketchup on the baby again.

It's a pushchair thing!

Pushchairs have their uses. You can carry your shopping in a pushchair, and you can't in a sling. But then you can always get a shopping trolley. They are cheaper, lighter and stronger than pushchairs and will be handy throughout your pregnancy as well.

If you go round to a friend's house with your baby in a pushchair, you can put her down in it when she falls asleep. Someone entering the room will think 'Oh, look, a baby' and take due care. If you park your sleeping baby on a bed, you'll have to hover nearby and remind people that that's actually a baby asleep there, not a large doll. Maybe your friend could hold her while she's asleep? People don't get enough chance to cuddle babies.

Once your baby is mobile, it can be handy to have something (other than yourself) to strap her to, to keep her still. It's not natural to tie your toddler into a wheeled chair to keep her safe, but then our world contains all sorts of unnatural dangers, like revolving doors and speeding traffic.

And finally, pregnancy and birth is not always kind to a woman's anatomy. Pubis symphysis or back pain can make baby carrying difficult or impossible. Hey, in that case, why not use that wonderful modern invention – the pushchair!

Out and about without your baby

OK, the time has come to separate that inseparable biological and social unit. Let's get busy with the breast pump.

- Read page 32 and pages 56 to 59 for the basic techniques for expressing milk.
- Sterilise all bottles, teats, lids, collection containers and breast pump parts. Use a steam steriliser, sterilising solution, or boil everything for ten minutes in a lidded pan.
- Try expressing milk from one breast while you feed from the other. It's likely to be dripping out anyway in the early days.
- Other good times to try are half an hour after a feed, or any time your breasts feel very full.
- Don't expect to get very much the first few times you try. Your breasts will eventually 'learn' to let the milk flow when you start pumping. One of my friends who uses an electric pump regularly has found that her milk gushes any time she walks past an electrical appliance which makes a low humming noise!
- You'll have more milk in the morning, so that can be a good time to try.
- Express directly into the storage bottle if you can. If you are going to freeze the milk, leave two centimetres of space at the top for it to expand.
- Label the bottle with the time and date of expressing.
- Store in the fridge at the back of the lowest shelves. Measure the temperature there. If it's 5-10°C use it within three days. If 0-4°C, use within eight days.
- Breastmilk that has been frozen doesn't have all the same properties as fresh breastmilk, but it's still very good for your baby. You will need to use a freezer, not the icebox of a fridge as breastmilk must be stored at -18°C or lower. Thaw in the fridge and use within 12 hours. Do not refreeze after thawing.
- If you need to thaw frozen breastmilk quickly, stand the bottle in hot water and use immediately.
- Don't use a microwave to heat or defrost breastmilk as it destroys the good qualities.

Some babies will switch happily between breast and bottle. Some won't. Some mothers really want their babies to be able to take bottles, so they start expressing and giving bottles when the baby is four or five weeks old. Other women practice total breastfeeding (see page 172) for the first six months for its contraceptive benefits, and don't try expressing milk until later.

If your baby is reluctant to take a bottle:
- Express or defrost a *small* amount of milk. You're going to have to throw it away if he doesn't take it, so just try with a little bit.
- Don't wait until he's screaming hungry or he'll just get cross that you've still got your bra done up. Don't sit in your breastfeeding chair or hold him in a breastfeeding position.
- If your partner is doing the bottle-feeding, drape one of your worn t-shirts over him so he smells milky to your baby.
- Smile at your baby, cuddle him, chat to him and let him gently explore the teat with his lips and gums. Make a game of it. Don't expect instant results.

Some breastfed babies just don't like bottles, and will go for a long time without eating. They really make up for it when you get home!

You don't have to stop breastfeeding when you return to work. It can be nice to keep providing perfect food for your baby all day, even if you can't physically be there with him. And the first breastfeed when you get home is a lovely time for you both to reconnect with each other.

Employers should support breastfeeding women in the workplace, because a breastfed baby is less likely to be ill, and his mother is less likely to have to take time off work to look after him.

Inform your boss ahead of time *in writing* that you will be breastfeeding when you come back. If they are aware of their obligations under the Management of Health and Safety at Work Regulations 1999 and the Employment Rights Act 1996 then they'll pop off and perform a risk assessment of your job using the European Commission Guidelines COM (2000) 466 final. Of course, you may need to remind them of this. Your work conditions have to be made compatible with breastfeeding.

You will probably need extra breaks, or shorter shifts so that you can breastfeed or express milk. Is it possible for your baby to be brought into the workplace to be fed? If not, you will need to use a private room to express milk. Preferably not the ladies toilet. Can your employer provide a fridge for storing expressed milk and a place to sterilise bottles? If that really isn't physically possible, you can use a freezer bag with ice packs to keep milk cool. Past a year, you may find that you don't need to express milk at work and can still feed your toddler in the evening.

If your job involves jetting off to foreign countries or, less glamorously, handling hazardous substances then it may be incompatible with breastfeeding. Night shifts, extremely stressful or physically demanding work might also be unsuitable – seek medical advice. If so, then you must be offered alternative work with the same pay and conditions. You should not be passed over for promotion or have your pay cut because you need to breastfeed. Let's not have to resort to a sex discrimination tribunal here! Men don't have to jump through all these hoops when they want healthy, clever breastfed babies.

So think through the practicalities ahead of time. You will need to express milk at roughly the same intervals that you feed your baby at home. Work out what you're going to need and discuss it all openly. If it will help, your GP and your health visitor can both write letters to support you in what you need to do.

Expect your milk supply to fluctuate. It'll probably drop a little by Friday, so have lots of snuggles and feeds over the weekend to bring your milk back on stream. If your supply seems to be failing completely, you can ask for your work conditions to be changed again to help it recover. If your baby suddenly refuses to breastfeed once you start work, then use the strategies for overcoming a nursing strike on page 183. Don't take on extra projects outside work. Don't expect too much of yourself. Consider co-sleeping, as it's a good way to keep up your milk supply. Be aware that your baby may become more clingy or start waking more at night. He loves you, and he is going to want more of you if you're away from him forty hours a week.

So you've sorted out the employer, you've got the super-duper hospital-grade expresso machine, you're prepared to break your back carting it into work on the daily commute, so now, what do you do with the baby?

Well, this is a touchy subject. Almost all mothers who return to work feel some degree of guilt about leaving their child. Usually it's economic necessity that forces a mother back to work, and although it's good to regain the status and social interaction that work provides, you don't want that to be at your child's expense.

If you can't do it, who's the best person to look after your baby? What about dad? That's a good option for some couples, but for many, it's the need for two incomes that has driven the mother back to work in the first place. Sometimes another family member can take on childcare, but our tax-credit system doesn't subsidise family-based childcare. Once the maternity leave has expired, mothers or relatives don't get paid by the Government to look after children. Professional childcare providers do.

So most parents have to choose between a childminder and a nursery. Now 'nursery' sounds like a lovely hothouse where children are nourished and watered and educated with all kind of stimulating activities. 'Childminder' on the other hand, brings to mind someone who will plonk your child in front of the telly all day. But often childminders are better for babies than nurseries. If we describe the options as 'individual' as opposed to 'institutional' childcare, we get an idea why.

Babies need loving, one-on-one attention. They need to know who to turn to to get their needs met, and that should be someone who knows them well, because they can't express their needs clearly. It's difficult for babies to get this in nurseries because they are cared for by a number of different people. Staff turnover is often high. Staff in nurseries tend to be more emotionally detached than childminders.[1] Very young children in full-time nursery care have higher cortisol levels.[2]

What if you can't avoid nursery care? Well, if it's for less than 12 hours a week,[3] you don't have to worry because scientists have found this level shows no measurable ill-effects. Attending the nursery with your child for a few days or even weeks can help him to feel comfortable there.[4] Take time every evening to connect with your baby – let him sleep longer in the day instead. And if you can choose a nursery that has enforced rest periods this will help his cortisol levels to stabilise,[5] which is actually better for an infant than masses of stimulating activities. Babies don't need education, they need loving interaction – it's personal attention which helps babies to develop language and reasoning skills. Nurseries with a lower staff turnover rate, more experienced workers and a lower adult to child ratio provide better quality care.[6] Unsurprisingly, these tend to be the most expensive ones.

These alarming observations only hold true in the early years when a child can't yet communicate easily. Once he's old enough to talk and to play excitedly with groups of children, then he'll probably love nursery. And if he doesn't, he'll be able to tell you about it himself. Some children are more sociable than others.

And even if you find the best alternative carer in the world, a young infant is still likely to cry piteously when you leave him. Because he loves you. Because you're well attached. Mine did. Oh, the irony of putting your child in childcare in order to write a book about parenting!

'You'll ruin your figure!'

Do you remember when you were a child, playing with your Barbie doll and thinking about what life would be like when you were Grown Up?

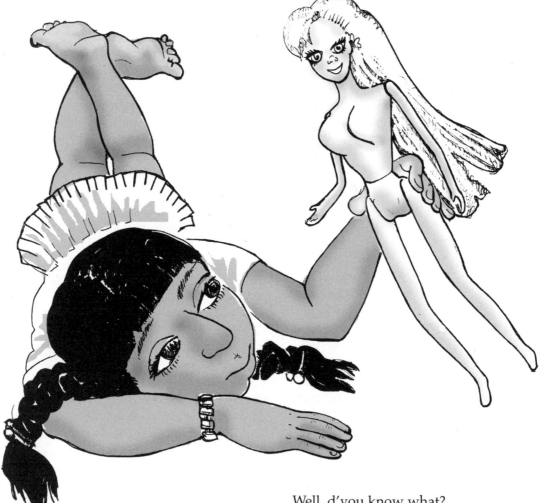

Well, d'you know what?
Real women don't look like that.

What do women actually look like?
Do we even know?

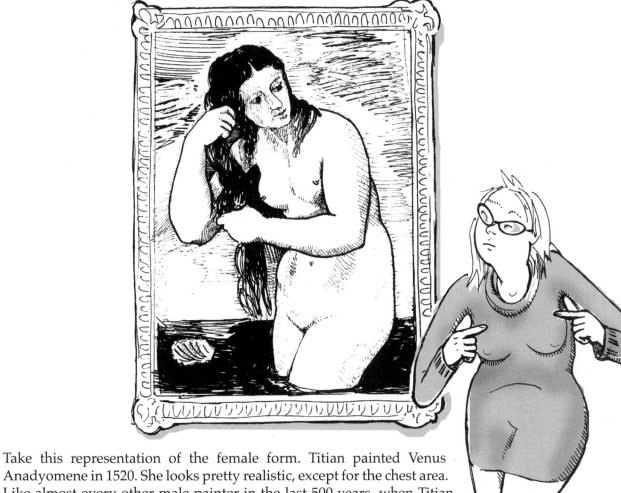

Take this representation of the female form. Titian painted Venus Anadyomene in 1520. She looks pretty realistic, except for the chest area. Like almost every other male painter in the last 500 years, when Titian painted breasts he took where the nipple is on the male torso (somewhere near the armpit) and he plonked a spherical mound behind it.

Breasts don't look like this.
The nipples normally hang considerably further south.

Really, I have to conclude that all these male painters never actually saw what women looked like without their corsets on, unless they were lying flat on their backs.

Of course, these days we have cameras. They give us a far more accurate image of the female physique. Not.

On the one hand, we see photos of giraffe-like supermodels, with their tiny, pointy breasts.

Of course, you don't look like them. You've just had a baby. Most of these women are too starved to ovulate.

Then there are glamour models. These women have large, round breasts. They also have very short arms and legs, and long torsos. So, when they stick their bottoms out, hold their stomachs in, inflate their rib cages and throw their shoulders back, their breasts look high-slung and perky.

You won't look like them either because you have to breathe out as well as in, round your shoulders and walk around doing normal human tasks.

You look like a normal human being.

My point is that well before women ever think about having a baby or growing older, most of us are concerned that our breasts are either Not Big Enough or Very Droopy. With no realistic images of the natural female form, we're all convinced that we're freaks.

And so girls go out and get themselves surgically remodelled, stuffed with silicone, sliced open and stitched up to meet some surgeon's idea of aesthetic perfection. Think about it – how freaky is that?

It's such a shame, because no matter how small your breasts are, you'll get your own natural breast enlargement when you fall pregnant. Three days after you've given birth, you'll have the most fantastic breasts. They'll be round, pert and disproportionately enormous. The reason why men find this attractive is that deep in their psyche they've clocked that this is the image of a fertile woman who can feed their offspring. Being sexy is meant to be linked to reproduction. Of course, at this point, sex will be the last thing on your mind.

So many women struggle with their altered body image after they've given birth, because the ideal we have of womanhood just isn't very womanly. We think we're meant to be thin, angular, uplifted, tight, flat and tanned. Now our bodies have done this most INCREDIBLE thing that women's bodies do, and we're dimp-led, streaky, wobbly, large, round and soft. And understandably worried that it's all downhill from here on the breast front.

Breastfeeding will not make your breasts droopy. Pregnancy might. Once they've got larger, they may not go back to being quite the same shape when they get smaller again. The shape of your breasts also depends on your weight and build and the stretchiness of your skin. Whether you have nineteen children or none, no-one is immune to gravity.

Mind you, it's a shame that low-slung breasts are so socially unacceptable, because they can actually be quite practical when it comes to feeding a baby. It's handy if you don't need to prop your baby up with pillows, and can just lie him in your lap. Maybe we're designed like this for a reason?

Why do we spend so much time being unhappy with the way that we look? Everyone does it. Those supermodels there feel too gawky, too tall and too flat-chested. The glamour girls are fretting about their short legs. It's time to start celebrating women in all the many shapes that we are. And to start valuing our bodies for more than the way that they look – for the amazing things they can do.

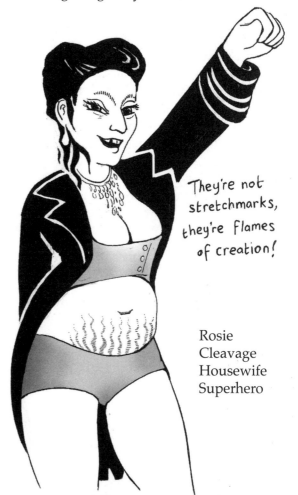

They're not stretchmarks, they're flames of creation!

Rosie
Cleavage
Housewife
Superhero

To bra or not to bra?

You know what else doesn't help with positive postnatal body image? Maternity bras. It is possible to buy funky maternity bras, and I could name-check Hot Milk, Bravado and Elle MacPherson at this point, but chances are your local bra shop won't stock them.

I suffered (really suffered) with first-week engorgement, so off I shuffled to Frome Ladies Bra Shop. This is a stalwart establishment which has been fitting farmers' wives with Supportive Underwear for the past sixty years. The lady there handed me an enormous white spandex garment with concrete interfacing and straps more commonly seen lacing up the sides of an articulated lorry. Team that monstrosity up with a pair of Caesarean-scar, waist-hugging granny pants and you have a passion-killing underwear ensemble that should never be seen on any woman under the age of seventy-five.

Some of the breastfeeding books I've read advise you to wear your bra constantly, day and night, presumably out of a fear that your breasts might droop if you don't. Well, I've tried not to generalise from my own experience when writing this book, but I didn't, and my breasts are fine. Skin-to-skin contact with your baby helps your breastfeeding, so I think you should spend time without a bra on, particularly at night. Just do whatever is most comfortable for you.

Assuming your breasts get large enough to need support after your baby is born, then your first bras should be comfortable. This is because pressure from tight bra cups can block your milk ducts and cause mastitis. Try taking a size up from the one you actually need – you can always sew up the straps later to shorten them. You don't have to buy nursing bras – soft stretchy ordinary bras can work well. If you do get one with lift-down cups, see if you can do the catch easily with one hand. Then get a couple the same, because it's less confusing if all your bras have the same mechanism.

Milky breasts are heavy. When the time comes to start taking exercise, you may want to team your bra up with a tight Lycra sports top to stop everything bouncing around.

Underwire is not recommended in the early months because it presses into the milk ducts. Fortunately, your milk supply will settle down in time, and you will become less susceptible to blocked ducts. If you've been feeding well for six months or so, you could try getting back into underwire bras. It's quite easy to breastfeed in a push-up bra – simply slip your breast out over the top of the cup. What's the point of having such an amazing cleavage if you can't show it off a little?

'Doesn't your husband mind?'

This chapter is written with a woman's partner in mind who, for the sake of argument, I will assume is male and refer to as 'dad'.

Well, dad, I owe you an apology. I have almost entirely failed to acknowledge your existence anywhere else in this book. All kinds of topics have been broached in which your vital role in babycare needs to be discussed, but nowhere have I written 'Now dad, do this and that, or such and such'.

There's a good reason for this. A proportion of fathers out there have little or no input whatsoever into the care of their children. And the mothers of those children are going to find it really irritating to read a book which says 'father can take the baby, while you have a break'. It's liable to make them collapse weeping on the floor yelling 'Chance would be a fine thing!'

Still, my oversight needs to be remedied, because your role in babycare can make or break the breastfeeding experience. But first, a word about how you might be feeling.

It's tough, isn't it? You meet a woman, fall in love, have a baby, and now she's in love with someone else. You'd better fall in love with him too. It won't necessarily be love at first sight – it might be a more gradual falling-in-love process. And you might struggle with feelings of redundancy and rejection along the way.

She's the one with the hormones. She's usually the one with the 'natural' bond with the baby. She's the one the baby yells for every time he's hungry, or tired, or hurt. You're the one he'll turn away from. She's the one he'll turn to.

And what happened to your relationship with her? Why can't you have a simple conversation for just ten minutes without her jumping up to check on the baby? Why is she so snappy? When will either of you get any sleep? Why doesn't she want to have sex any more? I mean, we don't want to rush things here, and you don't want to pressure her but hey, a man has URGES you know!

If back in early childhood you were dropped in your mother's affections when a new baby came along, then you might feel jealous of this new baby too.

Well, don't feel redundant. You can't breastfeed, but you can make breastfeeding happen. It's wrong that fathers are made to leave their partners and new babies in hospital in the precious first hours after birth. This new mother needs supportive nursing care for at least the first six weeks to get the time and energy to build up her milk supplies. If you cook, clean, tidy, wash up and launder then breastfeeding will go more smoothly. If, on the other hand, you spend your paternity leave on the sofa watching the football while your wife makes you sandwiches then you'll be worse than useless. Single mothers can ask people to help them. Women with unsupportive partners are worse off, because everyone will assume that they're getting some help and care, when they're not.

Your role doesn't have to be confined to housework either. Snuggle the baby on your bare chest. Skin-to-skin contact is nice for babies. He already knows your voice from the womb and now he can learn to be comforted by your feel and smell. Bathe him. Massage him. Try soothing him to sleep. It won't work every time because you don't have those magical bosoms, but if you keep at it, you'll find that some of the time it will. You superstar.

Take the baby whenever you can, so your partner can get some uninterrupted sleep. Expressing breastmilk could mean that you can feed your baby too, although this has implications for her fertility (see page 172). If you both want this to happen, you could take over sterilising and assembling the breastpump. That's one of those technical jobs that blokes tend to like.

It doesn't help your bond with your baby if your partner hovers over you criticising what you're doing. She's very, very wrapped up in this baby, and thinks she knows everything about what he likes best, but you need space to develop your way of doing things.

It will help your bond with your partner if you remind her of what an incredibly good job she's doing. She deserves comments like 'You're so good with him. I don't know how you do it!' 'You're amazing.' 'You're such a good mother.' With a few simple words you can transform a situation from one where she thinks she's reaching the end of her tether to one where she's walking on air.

She also probably thinks that she's not very sexy any more, and you're the best person to persuade her otherwise. I still can't promise that you'll actually get any sex. Sorry. If you start out with absolutely no expectations in this department, then you can only be pleasantly surprised.

In time you'll both slot into your complementary roles. You will find that you do some of the childcare better than your partner. Start out with general practical and technical support, then move into your specialist areas. Maybe you'll do the bath times. Maybe you'll do the bedtime stories. Maybe you'll bandage his scraped knees. Maybe you'll teach him to ride his bike. The more involved you are in childcare, the more rewarding it is.

The breastfeeding time can be tricky for dads. It is hurtful when your baby turns away from you for comfort. You need to be very big-hearted, and very far-sighted to see past that. Your baby will only be a baby for a year, but you'll be his dad for a lifetime.

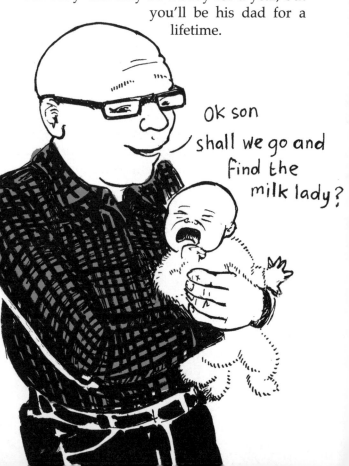

OK son shall we go and find the milk lady?

Sex and breastfeeding

Is breastfeeding sexy? This one confuses non-breastfeeders, because nipples are clearly an extremely sexually responsive area of the body. No it isn't. You can use your mouth for two different purposes – the nutritional one, eating food, or the sexual one, kissing. That's straightforward. It's the same with your breasts. The act of feeding a baby comes into its own, non-sexual mental category. There's nothing confusing about it.

Mind you, eating food is pleasurable in its own right, and so is dispensing it. Prolactin, the milk production hormone, is the same hormone that makes you feel relaxed after intercourse. Oxytocin, the hormone which lets the milk come down, is another feel-good chemical that is released when you make love. So every time you breastfeed, you get a little dose of the same pleasantly relaxed feeling that you might get after sex.

This tends to knock the edge off your sex drive. Your partner will feel an urge to make love to soothe away the tensions of life. You're already feeling physiologically relaxed, so that urge to dissipate tension isn't there. Also, breastfeeding suppresses your fertility, and you may not be aware of how much your sex drive is linked to ovulation. There is a point, usually about midway between their periods, when women feel incredibly randy and catch themselves eyeing up any potential mate that crosses their path. Men feel like this all the time! You'll probably miss that extra zing that ovulation used to give to your sex drive.

Do not be alarmed if you don't actively sexually desire your partner. This is only a temporary state of affairs.

Some people might see that as a reason not to breastfeed. That's only true if you view women as primarily important insofar as they are sexually available to men. There's a lot of pressure on women to be sexual beings – looking perfect, talking dirty, having effortless multiple orgasms like the women in the women's magazines. This isn't compatible with the pressures we face to be perfect mothers. None of us are perfect. Let's cut ourselves some slack here.

Getting multiple doses of feel-good hormones from breastfeeding is part of the sensual joy of being a woman. A holistic view of female sexuality recognises that women's sex drive and body shape are subject to flux and change as we move through different stages in our lives.

Anyway, it's not like those bottle-feeding couples are having nights of wild excitement either. Fatigue is an extremely effective passion-killer, for men too! Many women are psychologically traumatised after difficult births. And vaginal birth means that women have some physical healing to do. Get on it with those pelvic floor exercises, girl!

From an evolutionary perspective it makes absolutely no sense for a woman who has just given birth to rush out and engage in more sexual activity. Risking getting pregnant straight away would endanger the survival of the existing child. So women tend to be so psychologically wrapped up with their new babies that they have very little mental space for time with their partners.

This psychological link works both ways, too. Babies just seem to psychically know when you're trying to switch your attention away from them. At the moment when you pray

171

'Don't wake up right now!' they invariably do.

Caring for a new baby can leave you feeling so mauled, and touched, and crawled all over that when your partner leans over and starts pawing you too you just want to scream 'Everyone get your hands off me and give me some space!'

That was all the bad stuff about how babies kill your sex life. Now for some tips to overcome it. Just because it may not occur to you to initiate sex, doesn't mean you won't enjoy it once you start. Your sexual responsiveness is all still there – you just need a trigger to get started.

Now this isn't very romantic, I know, but put sex on your list of things to do. You'll already have a mental list that goes something like:

- Take those baby clothes back to the shop.
- Put the nappies on to soak.
- Cook the chicken before it goes off.
- Tax the car.

Add 'have a shag' to that list. That's the easiest way to make sure that you get round to it.

Last thing at night is probably not going to be your most passionate hour, because sleep will be infinitely more attractive than anything else at that point. Mornings could be better, but your baby may have other plans. How about when she goes to sleep at lunchtime, or in the afternoon? This is starting to seem even less spontaneous. Your list now reads: 'Have a shag – Saturday afternoon'.

Well, why not get a babysitter? I never could work out what else I'd need a babysitter for. I took my baby to parties, no problem. If we went out to a restaurant, we'd both rather he came along. But it would be really great to have a couple of hours to switch out of mother mode and back to sexy young maiden again.

If you are very good friends with another couple with a young baby, they may want to do a bit of reciprocal childcare for exactly the same reason. Not likely? You could ask a relative to take the baby while you 'iron out some relationship problems' with your partner, which is true, in a manner of speaking. Or you could get a babysitter to come to your house and then book into a hotel for the evening. Sordid, but exciting!

Use extra lubricant the first times you make love in case you are still tender. Caesarean or episiotomy scars can be painful, so you may have to try a different position. Sex is definitely the most enjoyable way to tone up your pelvic floor. Remember oxytocin = milk let down, so have a towel handy!

Breastfeeding as contraception

Total breastfeeding can help prevent you from becoming pregnant again, as long as you know the rules.

Total breastfeeding means meeting all your baby's needs for food and comfort at the breast. This means not regularly expressing milk for other people to feed, but responding to your baby directly. It also means not regularly leaving your baby for longer than three hours. Total breastfeeding means not trying to structure your baby's feeding and sleeping patterns. Total breastfeeding sounds like a nightmare if you think about it before you have a baby, but once she's here, it might seem natural and right (and difficult too, but that's what having a baby is like).

For the first six months of total breastfeeding it is unlikely, but not impossible, that your fertility will return. If it does, then you'll get a warning period first, before you ovulate. So the rule is, as long as you haven't had a period yet, you're safe for the first six months. If you do get a period, you have to use contraception from this point onwards. Lactational amenorrhea, as this method is known, is 98% effective. That's as good as the Pill.

After six months, the picture changes. Your fertility could still return at any time, but you could now sneakily ovulate *before* you get a period. The longer you go past six months, the more likely this is. This only happens for about 5% of women, but it does mean that it is possible to get pregnant again without ever having a period. Frequent breastfeeding will continue to suppress your fertility. Women who feed toddlers find that it takes an average of 14 months for their cycles to return, and some couples manage to adequately space their children using breastfeeding alone. But it's no longer a reliable form of contraception, so if you really want to avoid getting pregnant then use another method.

And, this isn't common, but if you are actively but unsuccessfully trying to conceive, then that can be a reason to cut down on breastfeeding or wean your child. Pregnancy tests are still accurate when you're breastfeeding.

The Pill and other hormonal contraceptives which contain oestrogen are likely to cause your milk supply to drop, so they are not recommended until your baby is older than six months and well-established on solids. If you have to use the morning-after pill, be prepared to spend some days trying to increase your milk supply again (see page 70). The mini-Pill does not usually affect milk supply but keep an eye on your baby's weight to be sure, and use the lowest effective dose. It can increase your risk of postnatal depression. Wait until your baby is six weeks old before taking hormones, so his kidneys and liver have a chance to mature.

IUDs can be inserted at the six-week postnatal check up. If you used a cap before, get it refitted as your cervix will have changed shape.

Co-sleeping as contraception

So the cot-death safety recommendations state that your baby should sleep in your room for a year. And this book says you should consider sleeping with your baby in your bed. Doesn't that mean that, er, how should I put this, activity of a sexual nature might occur near a sleeping infant? Is this psychologically harmful? Is it even legal?

They're asleep. It's fine. If they wake up, you stop. Just as you would stop if they woke up in another room, except you'll hear them more quickly and settle them back to sleep more easily. Presumably somewhere in their sleeping, subconscious brain they might store away some sounds that are associated with people being nice to each other. That's not going to do them any harm. Our society is rightfully concerned with the issue of child abuse, but children are harmed by violence, distrust, manipulation and fear, not by love, affection and respect.

Never mind whether it's safe, though, is having a baby in your room/bed/co-sleeping crib going to prove such a turn-off that it's a contraceptive in its own right? If so why not try making a love-nest somewhere else in the house? There's nothing like making out on the sofa to make you feel like a teenager again.

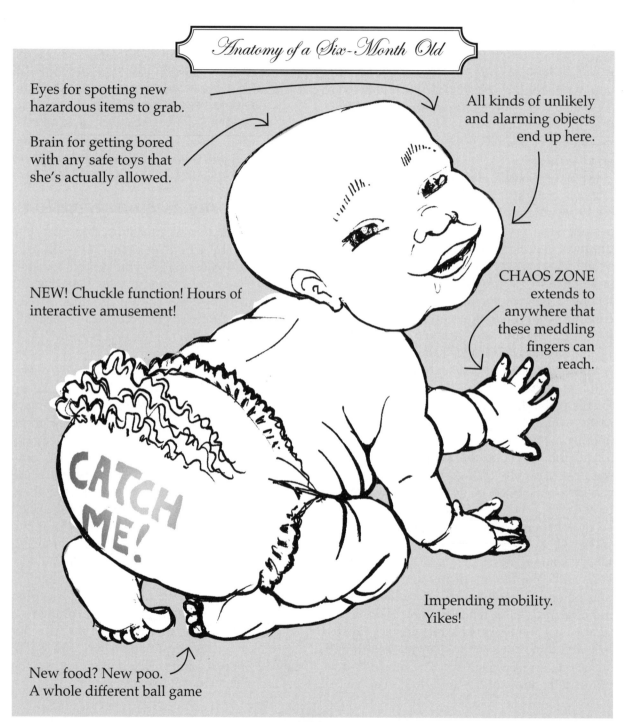

Eyes for spotting new hazardous items to grab.

Brain for getting bored with any safe toys that she's actually allowed.

All kinds of unlikely and alarming objects end up here.

NEW! Chuckle function! Hours of interactive amusement!

CHAOS ZONE extends to anywhere that these meddling fingers can reach.

CATCH ME!

Impending mobility. Yikes!

New food? New poo. A whole different ball game

Danger!

By six months, you will have received your free upgrade to the new interactive model of baby. Over the next few months she should develop into one of two basic models:

Happy Dumpling

This kind of infant will sit calmly on any surface, with no strong urge to throw herself off high places. You can sit dumpling baby on the kitchen counter while you cook dinner and she'll happily munch on a piece of fruit. When you find dumpling baby playing with an unsuitable item, you can peacefully substitute it with a safer one. If you have a dumpling baby, you can congratulate yourself on having such a chilled out, happy child. This must be, you assume, because you are such a chilled out, connected parent. It's not. All it proves is that you don't have a...

Wriggly Piglet

Once wriggly piglet achieves mobility, life becomes one long exercise in damage limitation. Marvel in wonder as she launches herself off three-foot drops, and keeps crawling! See how she can scale eight-foot ladders the moment your back is turned! Like dumpling baby, wriggly piglet is inexorably drawn to forbidden objects. Unlike her placid cousin, NOTHING ELSE WILL DO! and whatever strategy you employ to take the tin opener (for example) away then ABSOLUTE MELTDOWN will ensue. Teach wriggly piglet to swim and let her learn to climb. She's got some energy to burn off there.

As your baby's abilities increase, you will notice your own inexorable transformation into the Health and Safety Inspectorate's newest recruit. You'll become incredibly adept at spotting obscure hazards. This ability is particularly useful when you visit other people's homes. They won't notice that trailing lead that could bring a desk lamp crashing down onto your baby's head. You will spot it at fifty paces.

However, you're not going to discover the extent to which your baby can conduct herself safely unless you hold back and watch how she handles the common dangers that life throws at her.

Heights are a good example. Most babies will consciously stop at the edge of a sheer drop – scientists have tested this phenomenon by putting crawling babies in a room with half a glass floor. Some babies just seem to want to throw themselves off, just the once, to see what happens (humans are good at foolish curiosity). The point is that you aren't going to know which type of baby you have spawned unless you are willing to watch and find out.

If you grab your baby every time she crawls to the edge of the sofa then you've invented a brilliant new game where she'll repeatedly fling herself to the edge, just to get a reaction from you. One day you won't be watching. She'll get hurt. Because you tried to save her from the dangers of the drop, you prevented her from learning about it.

William Sears recommends *not* fitting stairgates in your home. This is based on years of observations as a paediatrician. Babies are harmed when they rattle stairgates that fail, catapulting them down the stairs, or when they scramble gleefully through the forbidden gate with no sense of the danger on the other side. A baby is not harmed if you teach him how to descend stairs safely (bottom first) and give him plenty of practice at it while he is still crawling and his centre of gravity is nice and low. You can still use stairgates if you want to, just bear these points in mind. This is all theoretical for me – our home isn't upmarket enough for stairs.

Take knives. Now obviously, you want to keep them out of reach of young children. But you also want them to know why. That means giving them a practical demonstration of what they do, where they are sharp and how they can hurt you. If you just issue a blanket 'This is Forbidden' command to a child without putting it in context you only make the prohibited item more attractive. A thoughtful child can learn to use a knife, axe, saw or hammer safely from quite a young age.

Be aware of the power of positive suggestion. If you hover over your child shrieking 'You'll fall! You'll fall!' somewhere deep in her subconscious she'll think 'Ah, Mum is telling me to fall here' and she will. Try to watch more calmly and observe while she learns to place her hands and feet. If you really can't do this, let Dad take over.

Fortunately one of the many superpowers that you attain with motherhood is a lightning-fast reflex when danger really threatens. This never fails to amaze me. I can't catch a ball. Not even from three feet away. But I can do a spectacular flying save on a toddler with a completely Jedi reaction time.

Some hazards kids can 'get'; some they can't. Sharp edges, drops and hot things have always been around; children learn to be aware of them. Toxic chemicals, electricity, speeding cars and broken glass are new hazards – our species doesn't have an evolutionary strategy to deal with them yet. So you do still need to be patrolling with that mental Health and Safety clipboard.

It's easier to trust your children if you trust yourself and your parenting. This is another area where tackling post-natal depression in women helps children. If you're depressed then your amygdala is hyperactive and imagined dangers seem very real to you, which means you can end up trying to wrap your child in cotton wool. While you can completely baby-proof your own home, depression can make it really stressful to take your child out to other more potentially hazardous households. So you end up staying in and missing out on social interaction, which makes your depression worse. This kind of nervousness can also make you think that your child is naughty when she is just engaged in normal risk-taking exploration, and that you are a failure when she does (as she will) get hurt. You're not.

Still, all mothers have different danger threshold levels. Some women are content to let their children run ahead on the street. Others insist that they hold their hand. And while many children can be trusted to stay on the pavement, a few think that it's funny to run in front of cars! There's no one right way to do this, just learn your child, trust yourself and be consistent with the levels that you set.

One other thing about risk-taking. Girls get stopped from doing things more than boys do, but when boys get hurt, they get comforted less than girls. Is it any wonder that women grow up with a limited view of their capabilities, or that so many men are emotionally distant and unable to process their own feelings? If you consciously decide to resist this ingrained sexist bias you will be helping to raise more whole and rounded human beings. So give your boys plenty of cuddles, and let your girls take a few knocks.

When it's time to wean

When is the right time to wean?

The word 'wean' has two meanings in English. It can refer to introducing solid food to your baby, or it can mean stopping breastfeeding. The first issue is more straightforward – when is the right time to introduce solid food?

A baby is born with an awareness of food. He's tuned in to your meal times, which is why he screams for a feed right at the moment you sit down to your dinner, and you end up having to eat one-handed while you breastfeed, and your partner has to cut up your steak for you.

It's also natural to want to share food with your baby, however, it's not natural for a young baby to eat it. That's why if you put it in his mouth, his tongue will push it right back out again. This is the tongue thrust reflex and it's there to protect him against starting to eat before he's ready.

Typical weaning advice for a four-month-old goes like this:
- Prop the baby in his highchair with special cushions.
- Sterilise your special baby-feeding bowl and special baby-feeding spoon.
- Open and heat or mix your packet of especially expensive baby food.
- Try to shovel the food into the baby.
- Watch as he spits it back out.
- Scrape it off his chin with the spoon and try again.

You're working against nature here. The baby's tongue, his gut and his immune system are all geared up to only need breastmilk for the first six months of life.

He might need quite a lot of breastmilk. Four months can be a time for a growth spurt that could have him feeding as often as a newborn baby. You might start to worry that your milk isn't enough for him. It almost certainly is. There are more calories in a teaspoon of breastmilk than there are in a teaspoon of baby rice, and it's more straightforward to get it into him. If your baby is thriving on your milk, then keep him on just that until he shows you that he's ready for something more.

Around six months of age, you will notice your baby watching you intently while you eat. If you let him, he'll pick up some food and put it to his mouth. The exact age varies with the infant. I knew one five-month-old who was clearly ready, lunging towards his dad's plate and grabbing a carrot. If your baby was premature or if he's had a significant gastrointestinal disorder then it may take him a bit longer. By this age (whenever it is!) his gut wall will have matured enough to handle new food proteins, his gut flora will be geared up to digest food better, his immune system is better developed so you don't have to sterilise everything and the tongue thrust reflex will have disappeared. All this makes the weaning process a lot simpler.
- Sit baby up in his highchair.
- Spread a mat out on the floor underneath it – things could get messy. (I had a dog for floor-cleaning duties, so I skipped this step).
- Put a lump of food in front of the baby. Anything that is bigger than his fist, and soft enough for him to be able to gum. A boiled potato. A bit of cooked carrot. Half a banana. Some melon (no seeds). You get the picture.
- See what he does. He might just lick it the first few times. Don't put it in his mouth for him – leave it to him to do the feeding.

- Finish your own dinner in peace, keeping an eye on your baby, mainly out of curiosity to see how much he can get down him before it all ends up on the floor.

This is known as baby-led weaning. It has some advantages over the usual method:
- It's easier because you don't have to mash anything, sterilise anything, spoon anything or really do anything. Except a lot of scrubbing clean afterwards.
- It puts the baby in charge of what and how much he eats. Because he stops when he feels full, he's less likely to get constipated in the short term. In the long term, it's good training for learning healthy adult eating habits.
- It helps him develop good hand/eye co-ordination.
- It is particularly good for babies who don't want to do things that you want them to do. (The 'Hey-Mum!-I'm-not-a-performing-monkey' syndrome). It can be a battle of wills to spoon feed this kind of baby, and easier to let him get on with it himself.

Baby-led weaning isn't the only way to wean a baby, but it's a good way. Disadvantages are that it's messier, it will initially take longer and isn't suitable for babies with delayed motor development. You may also feel an urge to buy and feed 'baby foods' because we're trained to associate shopping with happiness.

What sorts of foods can a baby feed himself?
- Start off with big chunks or batons of fruit or lightly cooked vegetables. Chewing on a cooked meaty bone can help him teethe while he gets some nutrition.
- After a while you can introduce sloppy food. Give him a spoon, and watch as he gets it into his mouth, and eyes, and hair. You can help him guide the spoon if you want.
- When that finger-and-thumb pincer grip gets more developed he can have smaller things like grapes and peas, or food cut into smaller cubes.
- Once your toddler gets molars you can progress onto harder foods and tougher cuts of meat.

As long as they are sitting upright, babies who feed themselves are less likely to choke than the spoon-fed because they learn to coordinate their chewing and swallowing at a natural pace. They will cough or gag from time to time to clear the mouth of food, which is fine. *You have to watch your child all the time he's eating* just in case.

Babies don't need any salt or sugar in their food. It might taste bland to you, but that's because you're used to lots of added salt and sugar. Plenty of salty, sugary foods are marketed as being for children, like cereals, processed cheeses and meats and flavoured yoghurts. Avoid them. Start reading labels.

Don't give your baby sweet foods as a reward for eating savoury foods. That's training him to think of savoury food as less pleasant than sweet. And give your baby sips of water with his meals rather than diluted juice – it's better for his teeth and you'll save a fortune. Cow's milk isn't suitable for a baby under the age of one, unless it has been cooked or processed into baby formula. Over the age of one, give him full-fat milk, not skimmed or semi-skimmed.

If you introduce new foods one at a time then you will be able to spot it if something doesn't agree with him. Anything that comes out into his nappy looking the same as it went in isn't good. Certain foods may make him grumpy or farty. If you wait a month before trying it again, he may be able to tolerate it better.

Allergic reactions and food intolerances may become apparent after your child has been eating a problem food for quite a while, so this isn't an exact science. Children can either refuse to eat a food that they are allergic to, or they can crave it, so no clues there either. If your baby develops persistent constipation or diarrhoea, reddened skin or eczema, asthma, glue ear, a permanently dripping nose or bad nappy rash, see if it will respond to a change in diet. Acidic foods like oranges and tomatoes may give him a sore bottom if he eats them regularly.

But be creative in what you let your baby eat. Your breastfed baby is already used to strong flavours coming through in your milk, so see what he makes of pickles, lemon, olive, strong cheese or even mild chilli. He will approach foods without prejudice when he's young so this is a good time to try him, before he develops into a picky toddler.

Baby-led weaning works best if you recognise that milk (breast or formula) is still the main source of nutrition for a baby under the age of one, and food is an entertaining voyage of exploration. If you're set on the goal of getting a certain amount of food into the baby to reduce his dependence on breastmilk, then you may be better off spooning it into him yourself.

Which brings us neatly on to the question of when should you stop breastfeeding your baby? And you won't find an answer to that in this book. There's only one person who can make that call, and that's you.

So, when is the right time to wean?

'It's simple,' says my friend Rosie (Housewife Superhero and Mother-of-Three). 'You breast-feed until it does your head in, and then you stop!' Once you've tried breastfeeding, whatever time you want or feel you need to stop, then you can.

You know, there's nothing wrong with formula milk. It doesn't protect your baby's immune system in the same way as breastmilk, and it's more difficult for him to digest, but as a source of nutrition, it's adequate. And for some mothers and babies, it ends up being a good option.

Breastfeeding can be wonderful, sensual and easy – that's why I think all women should try to breastfeed. But there are always going to be mothers and babies who find it difficult, and we should recognise that and support women in whatever way they choose to feed their babies.

Breastfeeding requires time and support. Some women never get the kind of care that they need to get their milk supply established. Others struggle with the unhelpful, under-mining attitudes of friends, family members or even medical professionals. None of that is their fault.

Remember the 'tricky babies' and 'tricky nipples' sections earlier in the book? There is practical advice there to help women recognise and tackle breastfeeding difficulties, but the fact remains that cleft palate, tongue-tie or low milk supply from breast surgery are real problems that can completely derail a woman's breastfeeding experience. Being faced with a baby who is screaming, fighting the breast and steadily losing weight, what other option does a woman have than to supplement with formula? She can add expressing milk to her 24-hour-a-day struggle to make breastfeeding work, and nursing supplementers are good if your baby will take them, but at what point does it all become too much?

Have you read the 'Common breastfeeding complaints' chapter? What if you were suffering from recurrent blocked ducts, which lead to mastitis, which lead to abscesses, which resulted in thrush from the antibiotics that you had to take? How far would you go with that cycle before you'd had all the pain that you could take? If you haven't been there, don't judge.

What about survivors of sexual abuse? Some women find that feeding their baby heals the trauma of breast-related assault. But others struggle with fundamental feelings of revulsion. That's not helping their loving bond with their baby, which is actually the most important thing.

In the old days, breastfeeding was often a shared experience. If your baby wasn't thriving then your sister, a friend or a hired wet nurse would help out. That's not a particularly socially acceptable solution these days. It's just you and your baby, and a lot of guilt, worry and intense social pressure to be the perfect mother.

If you want breastfeeding to work and it doesn't then that's horrible. No-one really understands. Your happy breastfeeding friends will be full of suggestions, but they don't know what it's like, because it was relatively easy for them. Your bottle-feeding friends will console you that 'formula is fine'. No-one acknowledges how incredibly hurtful it can be to feel that you have failed at something as fundamental to your womanhood as sustaining your baby with your own milk.

And if you have tried breastfeeding and you hate it, you're allowed to stop doing it. What is gained by telling a woman that she must suppress her feelings of irritation and dismay each time her child wants to feed? Let's forget successful breastfeeding and talk about successful mothering. That means doing those things, whatever they are, that make it easier for you to love your child and to parent in the way that you want to.

Mixed feeding

Exclusive breastfeeding to six months (or so) is best for your baby's digestion because his gut lining is 'leaky' with spaces that let food particles straight into his bloodstream. However, if breastfeeding is going so badly that you are considering giving it up, another option can be to mix breast and bottle. Your baby still gets comfort and immunity from breastmilk but you get a break from breastfeeding too.

- Your milk works on a supply and demand basis. That means that supplementing with formula will probably cause your milk production to drop. But it also means that as long as you put your baby to your breast, you will still make milk.
- Mixed feeding is going to work best if you exclusively breastfeed for at least six weeks, and preferably three months, before you introduce any bottles of formula. In the early months, your breasts are still 'learning' how to make milk efficiently. Starting formula supplements too soon could mean that they never get up to full steam.
- But, if you know you're going to do some bottle-feeding then you may want to try your baby in the early weeks using your

own expressed breastmilk. There is more about persuading a breastfed baby to take a bottle on page 161.

- Just drop one feed a day and see how you feel – that might be all the break you need. Wait a week before dropping any more, if you can help it, as this gives your milk supply time to adjust and stops you getting engorged.
- Watch to see that the formula milk agrees with your baby. Signs of allergic reaction are listed on pages 81 and 179. They can take some time to develop.
- Your baby won't be hungry for quite a while after a bottle of formula. This doesn't mean that your milk is no good, or that your milk is not enough for her. All it proves is that formula milk is more difficult to digest.
- I'm sure you don't want to hear this, but it's good to continue with some night feeds because levels of the breastfeeding hormone prolactin are higher at night. If you're really desperate for sleep, have one night off and then see if you feel better enough to feed again the next night. Maybe you could take it in turns with your partner? Try to nap in the daytime too.
- Co-sleeping goes well with mixed feeding. If your baby has a lot of access to your milk during the night then you can be reasonably sure that your supply won't suffer if she has a bottle during the day.
- Another way to keep up your milk supply is to have some skin-to-skin relaxed feeding time every day, in an evening bath for example.
- Don't top your baby up with formula after each breastfeed. She'll learn that she can get the milk quicker from a bottle and start to skip the breastfeeding stage.

How to feed formula milk

What you need to know:

Powdered formula milk is not sterile, and can contain disease-causing pathogens such as Enterobacter sakazakii, which causes vomiting, diarrohea, and even meningitis. Couple this with the fact that your baby isn't getting a protective dose of antibodies from breastmilk, and you can see why it is so important to be scrupulously careful when preparing feeds.

- Only use water that is 70 C or hotter to prepare feeds, which in practice means a kettle that is fresh off the boil. This is enough to kill any germs in the formula.
- Make up each bottle fresh each time you need one. Don't prepare bottles in advance and then reheat them, because this creates the conditions for germs to breed.
- Throw away any milk that your baby doesn't drink within an hour from when you made it.
- Always sterilise your equipment, keep work surfaces clean, and wash your hands before you start.

If you follow these rules every time, then any risk to your baby is reduced 10,000 fold. It also makes formula a lot less convenient and portable than breastfeeding. Sorry! We're following the World Health Organisation's latest research here. Shockingly, some formula manufacturers still advise that feeds can be prepared with cool boiled water or mineral water. It seems likely that they don't want to publicise the fact that there could be germs in the milk that they sell. See www.babymilkaction. org for more information about unsafe bottle feeding and its effects.

What you'll need:

- Some commercial baby milk. Don't give unmodified cow, goat or soya milk to babies under one. Goat milk baby formula has some claims to be closer in composition to human milk than cow based formula. Your health visitor can prescribe hypoallergenic formula for babies with allergies.
- Babies tend to drink about 150ml of milk per kg of body weight per day, or $2^1/_2$ oz per pound of weight if you still think in Imperial measures.
- You can buy a steam steriliser, a microwave steriliser, or use a large plastic container, with a lid, full of sterilising solution (follow the instructions carefully). Or you can boil everything for 10 minutes in a saucepan with a fitted lid. You can leave the lid on and let it cool, and it will remain sterile until you take the lid off.
- As well as a baby bottle with a lid, you need a sterilised flat plastic spatula or knife, and a bottle brush.

What you'll need to do:

- Wash everything well, including your hands and work surfaces. Use a bottle brush inside the bottle. Turn the teat inside out and scrub it with a little salt and washing-up liquid. Rinse everything thoroughly. Hang your bottle brush up to dry.
- Boil a large kettle of water and use it straight away. *It needs to be 70 C or hotter to be safe.*
- Take the bottle out of the steriliser. Don't rinse it or dry it, or touch the inside. Shake off the sterilising solution and put it down on the counter.
- Fill the bottle with the right amount of water. Check the level by getting down and looking at it at eye level.

- Put the right amount of powder in the water. Packing more powder into a bottle of formula will not make your baby less hungry, it will only make him fat. Dip the scoop provided into the powder, lift it up and then knock the extra powder off level with the back of the sterilised plastic knife. Don't squash the powder into the scoop with the knife or the side of the tin.
- Take a teat out of the steriliser by holding it by the edges. Shake off the sterilising fluid, but again don't rinse it or try to dry it or you'll unsterilise it. Put it on the bottle. Now get the ring and screw it on, then finally the lid.
- Shake the bottle lots to make sure all the powder has dissolved.
- Cool the bottle by running the base of it (not the teat end) under a cold tap. Shake some onto your wrist to check the temperature, and when it feels cool enough, use it straight away.

When it's time to feed:

- Whenever you can, feed your baby whenever she's hungry, just like with breastfeeding.
- Cuddle your baby fairly upright, look at her and chat to her while you feed her. Just like breastfeeding, this can be a special time for the two of you. You don't have to let anyone else feed your baby unless you want to.
- *Don't ever prop your baby up with a bottle* or leave her unattended while she feeds in case she chokes.
- Let your baby stop when she's full. Burp her. See if she wants a little more, but don't force her – she needs to be able to regulate her own appetite. *Throw away any milk that you don't use within an hour* because germs will begin to breed in it.
- Rinse out the teat and bottle after use.

Really, when is the right time to wean?

There is a common misperception in our society that because it's possible to get a four-month-old baby to take baby rice, then you should stop breastfeeding at this point. Like they've grown out of breastmilk by then. This is nuts. Women only just get their breastfeeding established when they start fretting about when they're going to stop.

The first few months of breastfeeding are the tricky bit. That's when your nipples crack and there's milk everywhere and the baby feeds for ages and you worry about his weight. But as your baby gets older it gets so much easier. His mouth gets bigger so he feeds more efficiently, and he latches on better, and you know what you're doing. And he's eating food anyway, so you can see that breastmilk is more than nutrition, it's special cuddles, and it's pudding, and it's keeping him safe from the bugs and the nasties that he can get now that he can go out and explore the world.

Your milk actually increases its anti-infective properties as your child gets older in response to all the new germs that he encounters. Once he's big enough to explore, he'll get bangs and bumps and bruises. It's nice to have the comfort of a quick breastfeed to soothe away the pain.

There is a clear medical case for continuing to breastfeed a baby well past four months. The World Health Organisation recommend that you continue to at least two years of age. I'm not saying that you have to do that – this is your choice. But if breastfeeding has settled down to the lovely, easy experience that it is for so many mothers and babies, then there's no reason for you to stop because *somebody else* thinks you should.

Don't decide ahead of time. Take each day as it comes. When you have a tiny baby then a nine-month-old seems like such an enormous fat piglet – you could never imagine still breastfeeding that! Motherhood is a hall of mirrors. Once it's your baby that's nine months old then he's just your perfect little man cub – those newborns seem strange and scrawny by comparison.

At some point either you or your infant will go off the idea. Actually, if your baby *suddenly* loses interest in breastfeeding, then technically that's not weaning. This is known as a **nursing strike** (which makes me think of picket lines outside hospitals, but I digress). Something has freaked him out and made him reluctant to feed. Weaning is a gradual, happy process whereas a nursing strike is a sudden, unhappy, absolute refusal of the breast. It can sometimes happen if you are separated from your baby for too long. It's not very nice for either of you.

- Keep trying to feed your baby. Try when he's not too hungry, when he's half asleep, lying down, or standing up, in the bath, somewhere quiet and without distractions, or while rocking or bouncing or singing to him. Something might work.
- Use a pump first so that there's milk right there and ready when he suckles.
- Try dripping milk into his mouth from a syringe while you hold him at your breast.
- If it has been a few days, try using a nursing supplementer, and express milk regularly to keep up your supply.

How to stop breastfeeding

You're here on the weaning page. Presumably you want to learn how to stop breastfeeding, and I just keep telling you new ways and reasons to continue. OK, so you've decided enough is enough. How do you stop?

'To wean' means to gradually reduce a dependence, slowly, by degrees. There is a reason for this. If you suddenly stop full breastfeeding overnight your breasts will become engorged like melons, you'll be dripping milk, in pain and at risk of blocked ducts and mastitis. But whether you manage to slowly, gradually stop breastfeeding also depends on how easy this process is for you and your baby.

With a very young baby, weaning can mean persuading her to take a sippy cup or bottle of formula milk. That's it. Gradually substitute bottles for feeds over a four-week period.

As a baby gets older, she'll probably become more aware that breastfeeding is emotionally meaningful. She may get upset if she can't feed, and might not be persuaded by a bottle. Some older babies will lose interest in breastfeeding once they start on solid foods, but they're in the minority. Most of them really, really like it and want to keep on doing it.

Some people see this increasing attachment as a reason not to breastfeed past six months. Some people think the opposite. Surely, the fact that a baby enjoys breastfeeding is a good reason to do it, quite apart from the health benefits? It's a natural, loving, physical relationship between a mother and a baby. That's a special thing.

Ultimately, how the mother feels about breastfeeding tends to determine how long she continues.

Three Stages of Breastfeeding Psychology

The First Stage: What am I doing? Ouch, this hurts! Everyone's telling me different things. Blimey, this is difficult. What if my baby starves to death?

The Second Stage: I reckon I've cracked it – breastfeeding, that is, not my nipples for a change. This is handy. This is cute. You want a snack baby? Sure!

The Third Stage: Are you not getting a little big for this? Blimey, I'm tired. Do we still have to do this? Wouldn't you prefer some juice instead? No? Really? OK, here it is.

You can be in the third stage for a while before you decide that it's time to stop. Sometimes a fixed date such as starting at work or college, for example, will galvanise a mother into bringing the breastfeeding relationship to a close.

Set out to drop one feed at a time over a few weeks. With daytime feeds, you'll be able to distract your baby. She might be more interested in food anyway, or an interesting activity can hold her attention. Rearrange the furniture so you can avoid sitting in your usual breastfeeding places, in fact don't sit down very much at all.

Sometimes dropping the daytime feeds gives a mother enough mental breathing space to carry on with night feeds for quite a lot longer. Other women find that it's the all-night snack bar that is impossible to maintain – they change their sleeping arrangements, but carry on with breastfeeds at breakfast and bedtime.

Dropping night feeds is difficult. Wear some impenetrable pyjamas, a bra and some heavy-duty breast pads. She'll be crying, you'll be dripping milk while you hold her, and you might be crying too. You will need to invent new ways of getting your child to sleep. Singing, swaying, carrying, driving, stories, music, bottles, dummies, anything that works, do it. If you can get your partner to hold your baby instead of you, then that can work well. Setting new sleeping habits is likely to take a lot of time and patience.

Once you've not breastfed for a few days, your milk will turn salty and unappetising, which can help complete the weaning process.

There is also the 'not recommended' method of weaning. This is where breastfeeding suddenly becomes ALL TOO MUCH for a woman and she abandons her baby with dad or with granny, and runs screaming to the hills. Baby will also be doing some screaming, although one advantage of this method is that after your baby has calmed down (which will probably take about three days) then it can really increase her bond with her dad. If you do this with a reliable, loving, familiar alternative carer then it's not bad for your baby. It is bad for your boobs.

If you deliberately or inadvertently end up in a sudden weaning situation then use a manual breast pump (not an electric one) to draw off just enough milk to make yourself comfortable. Express a little less each day. You can drink sage tea to reduce your milk production – make a strong brewed pot with two rounded teaspoons of the dried herb and drink three times a day, or more if required. Alcohol should theoretically help reduce your engorgement, so now might be a good time to go to the pub. Don't use either of these remedies if you are pregnant.

What if you don't want to wean?

How long should you breastfeed a child for? I'm sure you have an opinion on this. Most people do.

'You shouldn't breastfeed a baby once they get teeth.' But some babies are born with teeth. Does that mean those babies should never be fed at all? Why do you think they're called milk teeth? It's because they're the teeth they get when they're getting their milk.

'You shouldn't breastfeed a baby once they're old enough to ask for it.' Babies learn to ask for milk pretty quickly. You'll soon learn the special little grunt she gives when she's hungry. It's her first verbal communication with a specific meaning. Is that any reason to stop?

'But you have to stop before they get old enough to remember it.' Well, I know some people who can remember being breastfed, so I tested this one on them. What was breastfeeding like? 'Quite nice, actually.' 'Lovely and comforting.' They remember it fondly. What on earth is wrong with giving a child good memories of early childhood?

'You can't breastfeed if you get pregnant again.' You can. Many women choose to wean a child when they get pregnant because breastfeeding during pregnancy can be draining and difficult. Pregnant women often experience breast tenderness and reduced milk flow. But breastfeeding during pregnancy poses absolutely no risk to the developing baby, particularly in our well-nourished and cossetted society.

'Well in that case, you'll have to stop when the baby is born.' That's really going to help with the sibling rivalry isn't it? Move off the

breast there, it belongs to the new baby now. By contrast tandem nursing (as it's known) can be a lovely shared experience that strengthens family bonds. Once a new baby is born, your older child needs to know that she is still your baby too, and breastfeeding can reassure her of that. Tandem nursing is a difficult thing to do, but since there are good reasons for breastfeeding toddlers, some mothers decide not to deny their child breastmilk just because they have a younger sibling.

'But there are NO good reasons for breastfeeding toddlers!' Well, that's where you're wrong.

In 2002 the World Health Organisation decided that the case for breastfeeding toddlers was strong enough to make it recommended policy: *infants should be exclusively breastfed for the first six months of life to achieve optimal growth, development and health. Thereafter, to meet their evolving nutritional requirements, infants should receive nutritionally adequate and safe complementary foods while breastfeeding continues for up to two years of age or beyond.*[1] If every mother could do this, fewer babies would die. Simple as that.

Continuing to breastfeed keeps your child healthy. The immunoglobulin content of your milk after 20 months of breastfeeding is just as high as it was in the second week.[2] Breastfed toddlers are less ill, less often than weaned ones.[3] Some children are prone to recurrent infections or suffer from a long-term illnesses, and for them breastmilk is especially important. Other mothers choose to keep on breastfeeding because they are planning to travel abroad, where their child could be exposed to unfamiliar germs or insanitary conditions.

Breastmilk keeps on making your child smarter. Studies on the relationship between breastfeeding and IQ show that the longer you feed, the greater the difference.[4]

Breastfed toddlers are less likely to become obese than babies who are weaned in infancy.[5]

Breastmilk is food! People seem to forget this. If you think that children should drink cows' milk, then why not nutritionally superior breastmilk? A woman's milk *increases* in fat after a year, as her toddler burns off energy running around. A pint of breastmilk provides 30% of a two-year-old's energy requirements, a third of the calcium he needs, half his daily protein, 60% of his daily Vitamin C, three-quarters of his iron and vitamin A and 94% of his vitamin B12 requirements.[6]

'But it's not natural!' But it is! We're monkeys aren't we? If you extrapolate data from studies of primates, then we could be feeding our children up to the age of seven, which is when a child's immune system becomes as efficient as an adult's.[7] What we think of as 'natural' is usually culturally determined. Before industrialisation came along, Inuits weaned their children at seven, Hawaiians at five, Greenlanders at between three and four years of age and Aboriginal Australians between two and three years of age.[8] If you look at what we're designed to do, and what human cultures have historically done, then it's not particularly natural to stop feeding an infant when they still have an immunological and physiological need to suckle.

We think it's perfectly natural for a young child to suck their thumb or a dummy or nuzzle a special blanket or teddy. Breastfed toddlers generally don't need a transition object like this. What's more natural? To get your love and comfort from a human being or from a piece of cloth?

'It's weird!' It's not breastfeeding that's weird, it's our society. Breastfeeding past a year is unusual, so people don't know very much about it. When they see it, they tend to think 'Why is that mother making her child do that?' That would be weird, if a mother was trying to make her child into a little baby, and forcing him onto the breast. But that's not what's happening. You can't make a child breastfeed who doesn't want to – it's not physically possible. Sure, when you let a child breastfeed, you're letting him play baby for half an hour. You're his mum. He's allowed to be a baby. That's OK. This kind of continued emotional and physical availability helps a child to feel secure. When psychologists studied children who breastfed past a year they found they were really incredibly remarkably... independent![9]

'The mother must be getting something out of it.' This kind of accusation carries with it the assumption that because breasts are sexualised in our society, then breastfeeding must be vaguely incestuous. Believe me, there is absolutely nothing sexy about feeding a three-year-old. Women who feed toddlers are not always completely enthusiastic about it – it might often be easier for them to give the kid a drink of juice instead. Mothers do get something out of continuing to feed their children – they get smarter, healthier, happy children – but that's not to say that women always find it completely pleasant. They keep doing it because their circumstances make it possible, and they recognise that their child loves it.

The child must be getting something out of it. That's why he's doing it. When he stops wanting it, he'll wean himself. If you want to, you can just wait, and weaning will happen all by itself.

I'm not telling you how long to breastfeed for. All I'm saying is that whether you choose to wean, or to wait and let your child wean, that's nobody's business but your own.

Beat him when he sneezes

'And with that she began nursing her child again, singing a sort of lullaby
to it as she did so, and giving it a violent shake at the end of every line:
"Speak roughly to your little boy,
And beat him when he sneezes;
He only does it to annoy,
Because he knows it teases."'

Lewis Carroll, *Alice's Adventures in Wonderland*

You will, no doubt, have had plenty of opportunities to observe throughout the process of reading this book that the advice you receive here is at variance with other popular ideas you may encounter on how to bring up babies and young children. Really, you have my sympathy. Here you are, struggling through what may well be a sleep-deprived, relentless emotional and physical assault course, doing the multiple jobs that should be being performed by half a village, and you are surrounded by conflicting advice on how to do the single thing that's most important to you in the world.

'Don't let your baby cry' versus 'Let your baby cry it out.' 'Get that baby into a routine' versus 'Make sure you respond to your baby straight away'. There are two major schools of thought about baby-care in this culture, and they are completely at odds with each other. By definition, therefore, if you're 'succeeding' to raise your baby the way that one set of advice recommends, you'll be 'failing' to do it the way that the other side says you should.

And now I'm going to tell you that this doesn't end when your baby turns into a toddler, into a child, or even into a teenager. This fundamental, awkward, annoying schism carries on throughout the whole process of being a parent. You will always encounter people who disapprove of the way that you are raising your children, well after they're weaned.

I reckon the two conflicting philosophies of parenting can be summarised like this: **the child is meant to do what the parent wants and needs**, versus **the parent is meant to find out and respond to what the child wants and needs**.

This book falls squarely into the second camp. I think, frankly, that it's ludicrous to expect babies to follow a prescribed pattern of sleeping or eating (although I understand why parents want them to!). Babies need responsive parenting, and that means that their parents need to be actively caring for them, and wider society needs to be actively caring for those parents. The bonus is that when babies are fed and cuddled and tickled and played with 'on demand' they end up happier, smarter, sleep more soundly and become generally 'well behaved'.

'Isn't she a good baby?' strangers would comment to me and my bemused partner about our high-octane baby daughter. 'No, no, she really isn't!' we would reply. 'We just don't give her anything to get annoyed about EVER.'

I found this straightforward when my children were little babies. I didn't say I found it easy – it was insanely hard at times – but philosophically, it made sense to me. It also fitted into the pattern of parenting I'd seen in my own family. I'd helped raise a much younger baby sister when

I was a teenager, and she'd been breastfed on cue. (There's something very unsettling about disregarding your mum's advice when you make your parenting choices, but I digress.)

Anyway 'looking after baby' = 'do whatever they want', that's a simple equation. But what about when they get bigger? What about when your child starts to have more complicated wants and needs? Once they're old enough to explore the world? And get into trouble? And refuse to do what you say? And become *naughty*?

Well, we all know that if you spare the rod, you'll spoil the child. That children should be seen and not heard. You must teach the kid that 'no' always means 'no' or you'll be making a rod for your own back. Permissive parenting leads to children running wild! You don't want to end up with a spoilt brat! You have to show those kids who's boss!

There are parenting manuals on the market that advocate all kinds of tips and tricks to teach your child compliance with your every wish. There are star charts, and stickers, and button jars and bribes as the 'carrots'. Time-outs and naughty steps abound: banishment as punishment has tended to replace the actual sticks that our grandparents used to use.

This is not one of those parenting books.

So what's the alternative? We've all been lead to believe that if you're not a strict, inflexible disciplinarian, then you'll be an ineffective parent, some kind of wimpy, wishy-washy drip whose children will never listen to a word they say. But that's not true. There is another way.

Since we're discussing naughty behaviour, let's have a think about what that actually is.

Plenty of kids get into trouble for doing things that are normal and inevitable childhood behaviours. Running, jumping, screaming, spinning, acting the mad crazy fool, getting dirty, getting wet, blowing spit-bubbles, putting their hands in their pants – that's all normal for childhood. You don't have to tolerate it all the time in all situations. You can ask your children not to display the above behaviours, for example, at the dinner table. But allow some avenues for it some of the time if you want life to stay sweet.

I find a useful phrase to apply when judging when to restrict a child's behaviour is '**Why not?**' Children continually come up with novel ways to experience the world. Can they climb on the garden wall? Why not? Can they balance dog biscuits on the dog? Not right now because we have to catch a bus. Can they hit their brother with a rolling pin? Er, definitely not! The things that are absolutely forbidden are things that are dangerous and things that are mean. Everything else gets decided by negotiation.

So what do you do when they do the thing they're not allowed to do? I tell you what you don't do. *Don't get angry.*

It took me years to learn this one. The louder you shout, the less they hear. When you get angry with a child they freeze in fear and lose the ability to listen and to learn from the situation. If you don't want them to do this again, you want to them to pay attention. You need to be able to explain to them **why** this is **not**, not ever, what they should be doing.

I know anger isn't an emotion that's easy to switch off so you may need to employ a variety of strategies, but you're the one in charge of the discipline here, and that needs to start with yourself. Try counting to ten. Maybe you need some time out? Maybe you need some support and adult companionship? Parenting isn't meant to be a solitary occupation. Having said that, fear of being judged 'soft' by others often propels parents into being horribly harsh. Ignore everybody else's opinion right now. This is between you and your kid.

Find a way to communicate with your child. You may need to get down to their level, lay your hand on them and look directly into their eyes. You need at least two points of contact with a distracted, hyper kid. More if they've just eaten all the Halloween candy.

When a child does something dangerous it's simple to tell them 'don't do that because you'll hurt yourself' and explain the potential risks. What about when they hurt someone else? I want to create a world where deliberately hurting others is unacceptable. That's why I don't spank my children. And it's also illegal.

The first thing to do is to comfort the injured person. They are the ones who need the love and sympathy right away. When they're comforted, you can turn your attention to the aggressor.

Here's another useful phrase: '**Is it OK to hit someone?**' The child's eyes will either gleam with acknowledgement, or defiance:

'Yes, it is OK to hit someone.'

'Oh. So, is it OK for me to hit you then?' This only works if it's said in a spirit of calm scientific enquiry, not as an emotionally-charged threat. It's only acceptable if both parties know and trust each other. As a logical conclusion to this argument, I gently hit my daughter once. She stopped hitting her brother there and then.

If your child is too young to follow this level of argument then they're too young to be disciplined. Your job then is to distract them and prevent them from hurting others. You're not being 'soft', you're being age-appropriate. Giving everyone a drink of water is going to restore harmony a lot quicker than forcing a distraught toddler into the naughty corner.

Negotiating with children is a two-way process. Ask them for solutions – they'll surprise you. The best way to solve arguments between kids is to help them solve them themselves. Imposing a solution can result in everyone ending up dissatisfied.

The secret to successful discipline is empathy. However out-of-order your child has been, when they are crying, they are entitled to comfort. Yes, they need boundaries, but they must be loving ones. I know this goes against everything we've been taught in our society, but when a child is overwhelmed by extreme emotions, they deserve sympathy, not scorn.

Bad behaviour generally means that a child needs more food, more sleep, more exercise, less sugar or additives, and less screen time. Sometimes it's a reflection of your own bad behaviour. Once your child starts playing up, solving these underlying problems is a much more effective strategy than getting into a massive screaming confrontation. If you explain what you're doing, then you give them the tools to understand their behaviour: 'I'm feeling angry. Oh, but that's because I'm hungry!'

Calm, consistent evaluation and feedback is all that's required. You're in a strong position here, because you like each other.

Threatening children with punishments in order to get them to 'behave' is stunningly counter-productive, because the day will come when they will outgrow your ability to enforce them. Likewise, if you've trained them to unquestioningly obey instructions, watch out.

When they hit puberty, they won't be blindly following your orders any more, it'll be their peer group telling them what to do, and you won't have any control over the results. If, instead, you have always encouraged critical thinking then there's a slim chance that they'll engage their brain before following others into unwise escapades.

So, threats are out as a parenting tool. What about bribes? What about praise and positive reinforcement? We do have to make kids do things that they don't want to do. We have work to go to, and schools to attend, and trains to catch. Surely in that context, a sticker reward chart is no bad thing?

The strategy of praising children for good behaviour and ignoring bad behaviour is based on the theory of operant conditioning, developed by behavourial scientist B. F. Skinner. It was modelled on the behaviour of pigeons locked in boxes who had to press levers in order to receive food. Whether these theories should be taken and applied to child-raising is questionable.

Read *Unconditional Parenting* by Alfie Kohn. It's an excellent, original summary of the psychological research into rewards and punishments, the results of which surprised the scientists who were doing the studies.

The problem is that if you want a child to learn to do something, then they need to want to do it for its own sake. Take reading, for example. Reading is a pleasant activity. But when you create a school reward scheme for children to read books, they read shorter books, they don't understand them as well, and they become *less*, not *more* likely to read at home for pleasure. Study after study has confirmed this result. If you get your child to eat their broccoli by promising them ice-cream they'll learn that the vegetables are the unpleasant food.

Avoiding bribes and threats is intellectually challenging. It means being continually inventive. I had to reform my parenting, spot the points where I was resorting to bribery and think creatively about new ways to encourage and inspire my children. Mealtimes become an adventure with a giant eating an entire broccoli forest. Instead of stressing at a recalcitrant child to walk faster, maybe I could shout 'Tag! You're it!' and leg it down the street? Or sing a song with them? Or give them a piggyback? It's not like I ever get time to go to the gym.

This strategy really does bring its own rewards. Once they're old enough to participate in household chores, children are encouraged to take responsibility for their existence on more equal terms with adults. 'What do I get if I do the washing-up?' You get clean plates. You don't get a sticker or a tick or 10p. You get clean plates.

Raise your children with an empathetic understanding of their wants and needs. This is revolutionary parenting. It's about creating people who can think critically, not obedient drones. There will still be tantrums and tears, confrontations, but there will be a lot more love and laughter and mutual respect.

Nobody taught me this any of this when I had children. I shrieked. I yelled. I flung things. (OK, I still shriek and fling things sometimes, but I'm no longer under the illusion that it's acceptable or constructive). I stuck my kids in time out. I ignored them when they were naughty and praised them when they were good. I discovered the hard way that punitive parenting leads to stressed, depressed children.

So here, for free, learn from my mistakes.

Full-term breastfeeding for the fainthearted

I thought I'd wean my baby at three months. I was having a nightmare with a breast abscess, then I cracked the other nipple. 'That's it!' I thought and fed him a bottle of formula. Which disagreed with him so violently that I instantly changed my mind.

I decided not to wean at six months because everything was going smoothly by then. He was getting fat. We were on holiday. I didn't want to mess around with bottles. I thought I'd wait a bit.

At nine months, he caught a chest infection and needed some extra immune protection. I thought, 'There's no harm in waiting until a year.'

His first birthday came and went. We carried on breastfeeding. What kind of a birthday present would it have been to end something that he loved so much?

By this point all my friends who'd had babies at the same time as me had weaned. My friends who'd had babies since me had weaned. It was just me and him now. We were taking our first tentative steps (literally, for him) into the world of extended breastfeeding. We were on our own.

Actually, I don't like the phrase 'extended breastfeeding' because it kind of implies that the women who do it have extended breasts. (I don't, since you ask.) It's more accurate to describe feeding toddlers as 'natural term' or 'full-term' breastfeeding. I explained the medical, anthropological, sociological, physiological and nutritional rationale for feeding toddlers on pages 185 to 187. This section is concerned with the practicalities.

Breastfeeding toddlers can be lovely and cuddly and wonderful and incessant and demanding and exhausting. All at the same time. Referring back to the three stages of breastfeeding psychology on page 184, it's possible that the mother of any breastfeeding toddler might be in the third stage, the mildly irritated phase, for quite a lot of the time. Toddlers' demands are extreme, and just because you're basically committed to the breastfeeding situation doesn't mean that you'll always find it as delightful or convenient to breastfeed as your child will.

But really, it's not the child who is irritating if you breastfeed past a year, it's everyone else. You might encounter open disapproval if you breastfeed in public. Friends and family can directly question your mothering in quite a hurtful way. In a way, that's OK, because

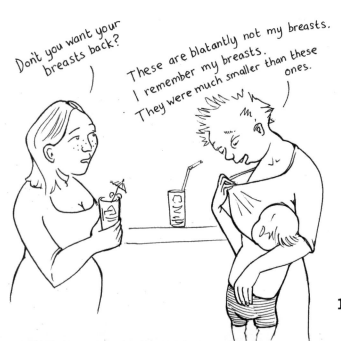

you can stand up to hostility. You can make a clear case for why continuing to breastfeed is in your child's best interests, and remind the concerned parties that since they are not the ones doing the breastfeeding, it's actually none of their business.

What's really annoying is that, because feeding toddlers is so rare, you're not likely to receive any kind of informed emotional support at all. Any time I ever expressed the slightest hint that I was finding breastfeeding difficult, the standard response was 'Why don't you just wean?' They always said 'just wean' – like it would 'just' be so damn simple. 'BECAUSE,' I felt like yelling, 'JUST because I'm feeling a bit PREMENSTRUAL and my breasts are a bit TENDER – THAT DOESN'T MEAN I WANT MY CHILD TO BE UTTERLY DISTRAUGHT AND SPEND THE NEXT THREE DAYS HOWLING ON THE FLOOR! I DON'T not want to do it THAT MUCH!!!'

I went to a La Leche League breastfeeding toddlers meeting. It was great. I haven't given La Leche League enough praise in this book, so I'd better slip some in at the end here. The name's a bit weird – it sounds like the Girl Guides with nursing bras – but the women there are brilliant. Anyway, I really liked the meeting. The mothers there were all so...

normal! I stopped feeling like a freak.

A couple of considerations for if and when you foray into full-term breastfeeding. Once your child is old enough to speak, he'll be able to ask for milk by name. One approach to this situation is to adopt a code word for breastmilk, to avoid embarrassment – 'bitty', for example. I dunno, I thought that was a bit twee. We used the word 'babymilk' because that's what it is. It also enabled me to exert just a little psychological pressure on my child to hurry up and self-wean:

six down 'to refresh or recharge'

'This is *babymilk*. It's for *babies*, isn't it?'

'Yes.'

'You're not a baby, are you?'

'Yes I am. I am a baby.'

As you can see, he was immune to my devious machinations. He knows his own mind. Good boy!

Although toddlers can feed a lot more quickly than a small baby, they may still want to breastfeed frequently, particularly at times of psychological upheaval. A common way of dealing with this is to adopt a policy of 'don't offer – don't refuse'. That way you're giving your child every opportunity to lose interest in breastfeeding if he wants to.

Some mothers impose restrictions on when or where their toddlers can breastfeed. Feeding in public is one which many mothers ban early on. Which is a shame really, because if more women were seen doing it, then more women would feel confident to do it.

You can train your child to request to feed politely. You can try to persuade him not to hurt you by wriggling around with those bony knees and elbows while he feeds. Breastfeeding toddlers can get incredibly acrobatic!

Consider the advantages of feeding toddlers too. They're amazingly good at investigating, and exploring, and running, and jumping, and swinging and...falling over! Breastfeeding can calm a hurt child so quickly and completely that it's a wonderful mothering tool.

It makes a real difference if you can breastfeed a toddler who's ill. Suddenly, your milk might be the only nutrition he can ingest. This miracle fluid can help to quickly clear up an infection that could otherwise be quite serious for one so small.

And breastfeeding a toddler can be very convenient. He might have a need to calmly connect with his mother. You might have a need to spend a while on Facebook. Stick the breastfeeding chair in front of the computer and voilà! we have a picture of family harmony.

I thought I'd let my child wean himself in his own time. Natural-term breastfeeding sounded like a good thing to aspire to. Then suddenly, something changed. I looked at my child as he was feeding to sleep and I realised that it was time to wean.

The mixed feelings didn't end there. It's a funny old world. You're doing it, and you may be not entirely sure that you want to, but it comes time to stop and you realise that you'll miss it like hell! The first thing that you did with your baby was put him to your breast – will he still be your baby if you stop? Will he still love you if you don't breastfeed? If anyone out there is struggling with the same feelings, be reassured, because I tested this, and the answers are yes and yes.

Once a child has a good understanding of language you may be able to talk him into a calm and easy weaning. You can use reason – 'It's hurting mummy so we have to stop'. You can use peer pressure – 'Your friends don't feed because it's a baby thing.' You can fib a little – 'There's none left – it ran out!' If it comes to it you can use bribery – maybe a big Weaning Day celebration will do the trick? And as with younger babies you can use substitution and distraction – a sippy cup of rice milk and about eighteen bedtime stories worked instead of breastfeeding to get my son to sleep.

Don't forget that after a four-day break (a holiday with dad?) your milk will turn salty. 'It's gone off, just like the milk in the fridge does' should appeal to a young child's sense of logic.

Many children can lose interest in breast-feeding before mothers feel they need to impose weaning. From the crawling baby who pushes away the breast and reaches for a banana to the four-year-old who announces that she's stopped because she's a Big Girl now – they've all reached the end of their own individual natural term.

The breastfeeding chapter of mothering has ended. It's time to turn over to a new page.

Sources and resources

If you are having difficulty breastfeeding then the personal advice of a breastfeeding professional is invaluable. That's a lactation consultant. Not a doctor, or a nurse, or a health visitor (although they can be good too). Ask to be put in touch with one through your midwifery practice. The La Leche League, the National Childbirth Trust and the Association of Breastfeeding Mothers all provide trained counsellors to help you in your hour of need. For online breastfeeding information, www. kelly mom.com and www.asklenore.info are good places to start a web search.

Recommended further reading on breastfeeding:

Ina May's Guide to Breastfeeding by Ina May Gaskin (Pinter & Martin, 2009). Just excellent. Plenty of practical advice for complaints and modifying problem behaviours. She also discusses 'nipplephobia' in society, and the practical value of cross-feeding.

Breastfeeding Special Care Babies by Sandra Lang (Bailliere Tindall, 2002). Excellently written, practical and informative, with plenty of relevance for breastfeeding any baby.

Mothering Multiples by Karen Kerkhoff Gromada (La Leche League International, 2007). Another good all-round book on breastfeeding which is required reading if you give birth to more than one baby at once.

Mothering Your Nursing Toddler by Norma Jane Bumgarner (what a name!) (La Leche League International, 2000) is a reassuring read if you breastfeed past a year.

Fresh Milk: The Secret Life of Breasts by Fiona Giles (Simon & Schuster, 2003). A whimsical and brilliantly written series of essays on all aspects of lactation.

The Politics of Breastfeeding by Gabrielle Palmer (Pinter & Martin, 2008). Be inspired and outraged.

Of all the scientific studies I read while researching this book, I found 'Mental health, attachment and breastfeeding: implications for adopted children and their mothers', K Gribble, *International Breastfeeding Journal* 2006 to be extremely touching.

on babycare:

The Baby Book by William and Martha Sears (Harper Thorsons, 2005). Comprehensive, practical and baby-centred with the kind of medical authority that you can use in arguments with your mother-in-law.

Understanding your Crying Baby by Sheila Kitzinger (Carroll & Brown, 2005) will counteract all the terrible advice you'll receive if your baby cries a lot.

on sleep:

Willam and Martha Sears' *Baby Sleep Book* (Harper Thorsons, 2005) has a lot of practical suggestions for different ways to help a child to sleep.

The No-Cry Sleep Solution by Elizabeth Pantley (McGraw Hill, 2002) comes recommended as an alternative to controlled crying sleep-training regimes.

Three in a Bed by Deborah Jackson (Bloomsbury, 2003). A seminal work on co-sleeping, which has helped achieve a cultural shift on attitudes to infant sleep in today's society.

on mental health:

Healing Without Freud or Prozac by David Servan-Schreiber (Rodale, 2005) gives clear and effective advice for tackling depression and approaching life in an emotionally healthy way.

on the psychology of parenting:

Why Love Matters by Sue Gerhardt (Brunner-Routledge, 2004). An important and accessible work on how loving relationships underpin infant development, impressively researched with a thorough explanation of the psychology and neurochemistry involved.

Becoming Attached: First Relationships and How They Shape Our Capacity to Love by Robert Karen (OUP, 1998). A fascinating and very readable explanation of attachment theory.

What Mothers Do by Naomi Stadlen (Piatkus, 2005). An original, non-judgemental and extremely perceptive analysis of what the job of mothering actually entails. It will almost certainly increase your confidence in whatever you are doing with your children.

Frontispiece

page 2 (1) Infant Feeding Survey 2000 UK Department of Health

What are breasts?

page 8 (1) Ford and Beach 1951 quoted in *Breastfeeding: Biocultural Perspectives* by Patricia Stuart-Macadam and Katherine A Dettwyler (Aldine de Gruyter, 1995) p180

What's so special about breastmilk anyway?

page 19 (1) Breast feeding and obesity: cross sectional study. R von Kries, B Koletzko, T Sauerwald, E von Mutius, D Barnert, V Grunert, H von Voss. *British Medical Journal (BMJ)*, 1999: 319: 147-150

page 20 (2) Breastfeeding effects on intelligence quotient in 4- and 11-year-old children. SW Jacobson, LM Chiodo, JL Jacobson. *Pediatrics*, May 1999: 103: 5: e71 **also:** Breast milk feeding and cognitive ability at 7-8 years. LJ Horwood, BA Darlowb, N Mogridge. *Archives of Disease in Childhood*, January 2001: 84: F23-F27 **also:** The association between duration of breastfeeding and adult intelligence. EL Mortensen, KF Michaelsen, SA Sanders, JM Reinisch. *Journal of the American Medical Association*, 2002: 287: 2365-2371 **also:** Breastfeeding and cognitive function bibliography. Marsha Walker. www.naba-breastfeeding.org

page 21 (3) Presence of delta-sleep-inducing peptide-like material in human milk. MV Graf, CA Hunter and AJ Kastin. *Journal of Clinical Endocrinology & Metabolism*: 59: 127-132

page 22 (4) *Ear infections, urinary tract infections, allergies, cot death* UNICEF Baby Friendly Initiative. www.babyfriendly.org.uk *colds, chest infections, tummy upsets* Quantifying the benefits of breastfeeding: a summary of the evidence. N Leon-Cava, C Lutter, J Ross, L Martin. US Agency for International Development, 2002 *blood pressure* Early nutrition inpreterm infants and later blood pressure: Two cohorts after randomised trials. A Singhal, TJ Cole, A Lucas. *Lancet*, 2001: 357: 413-9 *heart disease* Breastfeeding during infancy and the risk of cardiovascular disease in adulthood. J W Rich-Edwards, MJ Stampfer, JE Manson et al. *Epidemiology*, September 2004: 15(5):550-556 *diabetes* 'Formula diabetes?' *New Scientist*, 10 May 2008 *straighter teeth and clearer speech* The relationship of breastfeeding to oral development and dental concerns. KM Westover, MK DiLoreto, TR Shearer. *ASDC Journal of Dentistry for Children*, March–April 1989: 56(2):140-3 *eyesight* Infant nutrition and stereoacuity at age 4–6 years. A Singhal et al. *American Journal of Clinical Nutrition*, January 2007: 85: 152-9

page 23 (5) UNICEF Baby Friendly Initiative www.babyfriendly.org.uk **also:** Quantifying the benefits of breastfeeding: a summary of the evidence. N Leon-Cava, C Lutter, J Ross, L Martin. US Agency for International Development, 2002

First feeds

page 44 (1) Labor pain effects on colostral milk beta-endorphin concentrations of lactating mothers. V Zanardoa et al. *Biology of the Neonate*, 2001: 79:87-90

page 50 (2) Lactation failure due to insufficient glandular development of the breast. MR Neifert, JM Seacat, WE Jobe. *Pediatrics*, November 1985: No. 76, Issue 5, pp. 823-8

page 51 (3) Mental health, attachment and breastfeeding: implications for adopted children and their mothers. K Gribble. *International Breastfeeding Journal*, 2006

page 60 (4) *develop better and go home sooner* Implications of kangaroo care for growth and development in preterm infants. VL Dodd. *Journal of Obstetric, Gynecologic, & Neonatal Nursing* 34 (2): 218–232. *lowered morbidity, sleep, breathing, heart rate, temperature* Kangaroo mother care – a review. D Hall, G Kirsten. *Transfusion Medicine*, 2008: 18:77-82 *pain and stress* Kangaroo mother care diminishes pain from heel lance in very preterm neonates: a cross-over trial. CC Johnston, F Filion, M Campbell-Yeo et al. *BMC Pediatrics*, 2008: 8:13

Oops, I appear to have too much milk!

page 77 (1) Overabundant milk supply: an alternative way to intervene by full drainage and block feeding. CGA van Veldhuizen-Staas. *International Breastfeeding Journal*, 2007: 2:11

How often should you feed yourself?

page 78 (1) Breastmilk calcium concentrations during prolonged lactation in British and rural Gambian mothers. MA Laskey, A Prentice, J Shaw, T Zachou, SM Ceesay. *Acta Paediatrica Scandinavia*, 1990: 79: 507-512

page 79 (2) Alcohol use during lactation: effects on the mother and the breastfeeding infant. JA Menella. Nutrition and Alcohol: Linking Nutrient Interactions and Dietary Intake. CRC Press, 2004. **(3)** Effects of exposure to alcohol in mother's milk on infant sleep. JA Menella, C J Gerrish. *Pediatrics*, May 1998: 101 : 5. **(4)** Maternal alcohol use during breastfeeding and infant mental and motor development at one year. RE Little, KW Anderson, CH Ervin et al. *The New England Journal of Medicine*, August 1989: 321: 425-430. **(5)** Alcohol levels in Chinese mothers after consumption of alcoholic diet during postpartum "doing the month" ritual. YC Chien, JF Liu, YJ Huang et al. *Alcohol*, 2005: 37:143-50. **(6)** Alcohol use during lactation: the folklore versus the science. JA Menella. *Current Issues in Clinical Lactation*, 2002. **(7)** Evidence of genetic predisposition to alcoholic cirrhosis and psychosis: twin concordances for alcoholism and its biological end points by zygosity among male veterans. Z Hrubec, GS Omenn. *Alcohol, Clinical and Experimental Research*, Spring 1981: 5: 207-15. **(8)** The transfer of alcohol into human milk: sensory implications and effects on mother-infant interaction. JA Menella. *Alcohol and Alcoholism: Effects on Brain Development*, 1999

page 80 (9) Maternal marijuana use during lactation and infant development at one year. SJ Astley, RE Little. *Neurotoxicol Teratol*, March-April 1990: 12: 2: 161-8. **(10)** Growth and pubertal milestones during adolescence in offspring prenatally exposed to cigarettes and marijuana. PA Fried, DS James and B Watkinson. *Neurotoxicology and Teratology*, October 2001: 23: 5: 431-436. **(11)** Passive smoking and sudden infant death syndrome: review of the epidemiological evidence HR Anderson, DG Cook. *Thorax*, 1997: 52: 1003-1009. **(12)** Tobacco and children. An economic evaluation of the medical effects of parental smoking. CA Aligne, J J Stoddard. *Archives of Pediatrics and Adolescent Medicine*, July 1997: 151: 7. **(13)** Risks and benefits of nicotine to aid smoking cessation in pregnancy. D Dempsey, NL Benowitz. *Drug Safety*, 2001: 24: 4: 277-322. **(14)** Smoking hygiene: an educational intervention to reduce respiratory symptoms in breastfeeding infants exposed to tobacco. KR Pulley, MB Flanders-Stepans. *The Journal of Perinatal Education*, summer 2002: 11: 3: 28–37. **(15)** Newborns who confuse night and day. S Mize. La Leche League International. *New Beginnings*, January 1995: 12:1: 14-15

page 81 (16) Effect of a low-allergen maternal diet on colic among breastfed infants: a randomized, controlled trial DJ Hill, N Roy, RG Heine et al. *Pediatrics*, November 2005: 116: 5: e709-e715

How often should you feed your baby?

page 92 (1) Menopause sets us apart from chimps. *New Scientist*, 22 December 2007 reporting research by Melissa Emery Thompson at Harvard University. The conclusion that post-menopausal women are socially necessary primarily for childcare is mine, not Emery Thompson's.

page 94 (2) Infant crying and sleeping in London, Copenhagen and when parents adopt a 'proximal' form of care. I St James-Roberts, M Alvarez, E Csipke et al. *Pediatrics*, June 2006: 117: 6: e1146-e1155

page 95 (3) This overview of attachment theory is informed by reading *Becoming Attached: First Relationships and How They Shape Our Capacity to Love* by Robert Karen (Oxford University Press, 1998)

page 96 (4) *US statistics*: Breastfeeding, Sensitivity and Attachment. JR Britton, HL Britton, V Gronwaldt. *Pediatrics*, November 2006: 118: 5: e1436-e1443 **UK statistics:** What is attachment? Child And Adolescent Mental Health Services Cambridgeshire And Peterborough Mental Health Partnership NHS Trust. www.camhs.cambsmh.nhs.uk

Night feedzzz

page 105 (1) International Child Care Practices Study: infant sleeping environment. EA Nelson, BJ Taylor, A Jenik et al. *Early Human Development*, April 2001: 62: 1: 43-55. **(2)** ibid. **(3)** Sudden infant death syndrome: links with infant care practices. M Gantley, D P

Davies, A Murcott. *BMJ*, 2 January 1993: 306(6869): 16–20. **(4)** Sudden Infant Death Syndrome among Asians in California. Grether JK, Schulman J, Croen LA. *The Journal of Pediatrics*, 1990: 116: 525-528

page 106 (5) Maternal proximity and infant CO_2 environment during bedsharing and possible implications for SIDS research. S Mosko, C Richard, JMS Drummond, D Mukai. *American Journal of Physical Anthropology*: 103: 3: 315 - 328. **(6)** and **(9)** *Baby Sleep Book* by William and Martha Sears (Harper Thorsons, 2005) p105. **(7)** and **(8)** Infant arousals during mother-infant bed sharing: implications for infant sleep and Sudden Infant Death Syndrome. S Mosko, C Richard, J McKenna. *Pediatrics*, November 1997: 100: 5: 841-849. **(10)** Why babies should never sleep alone: A review of the co-sleeping controversy in relation to SIDS, bedsharing and breastfeeding. J McKenna, T Dade. *Paediatric Respiratory Reviews*, 2005: 6: 134-152. **(11)** *formula-fed babies are 31% more likely to die of SIDS* Risk factors for sudden infant death syndrome following the prevention campaign in New Zealand: a prospective study. E. Mitchell et al. *Pediatrics* (New Zealand), November 1997: 100: 5: 835-40. **also** Comparison of evoked arousability in breast and formula fed infants. R S C Horne, P M Parslow, D Ferens et al. *Archives of Disease in Childhood*, 2004: 89: 22-25. **(12)** Differences in infant and parent behaviours during routine bed sharing compared with cot sleeping in the home setting. SA Baddock, BC Galland, DPG Bolton et al. *Pediatrics*, May 2006: 117:5: 1599-1607. **(13)** Bed sharing, breastfeeding and parental choice. HL Ball. Parent-Infant Sleep Lab. Department of Anthropology. University of Durham

page 107 (14) Manchester NHS safe sleeping practice for infants. **(15)** Babies sleeping with parents: case-control study of factors influencing the risk of the sudden infant death syndrome. PS Blair, PJ Fleming, IJ Smith et al. *BMJ*, December 1999: 319:1457-1462. **(16) (17) (18) (19)** Confidential Enquiry into Stillbirths and Deaths in Infancy, 3rd Annual Report, January-December 1994 (Department of Health, 1996) quoted in The Politics of Cot Death, *AIMS Journal*, winter 2003: vol 15, no 4

page 108 (20) Babies sleeping with parents: case-control study of factors influencing the risk of the sudden infant death syndrome. PS Blair, IJ Smith, M Ward Platt et al. *BMJ*, December 1999: 319: 1457-1462.

page 109 (21) Why babies should never sleep alone: A review of the co-sleeping controversy in relation to SIDS, bedsharing and breastfeeding. J McKenna, T Dade. *Paediatric Respiratory Reviews*, 2005: 6: 134-152. McKenna quotes a number of psychiatric studies of adults who co-slept as infants, including a large scale survey: The Effects of Childhood Cosleeping On Later Life Development 1998, a masters thesis by J Mosenkis, University of Chicago, Department of Human Development

page 112 (22) *Baby Sleep Book* by William and Martha Sears (Harper Thorsons, 2005) p103

Stress and depression

page 115 (1) The basic information on depression in this chapter was informed by a MindFields Seminar 'Effective brief therapy for depression' taught by Joe Griffin.

page 116 (2) 'Postnatal depression' Royal College of Psychiatrists' Public Education Editorial Board, August 2007. **(3)** indicated from correspondence with her daughter quoted in *Life After Birth* by Kate Figes (Penguin, 1998) p24

page 119 (4) *Healing without Freud or Prozac* by David Servan-Schreiber (Rodale, 2005)

page 122 (5) *Why Love Matters* by Sue Gerhardt (Brunner-Routledge, 2004) p68. **(6)** Postnatal depression and antidepressant medication and breastfeeding. W Jones. The Breastfeeding Network. www.breastfeedingnetwork.org.uk

page 123 (7) and **(10)** Acupuncture, exercise and fish oil supplements are three of the main recommendations in David Servan-Schreiber's book *Healing Without Freud or Prozac*. **(8)** St John's Wort for depression – an overview and meta-analysis of randomised clinical trials. K Linde, G Ramirez, CD Mulrow et al. *BMJ*, August 1996: 313: 253-258. **(9)** Interactions between herbal medicines and prescribed drugs: a systematic review. AA Izzo, E Edzard. *Drugs*, 2001: 61: 15: 2163-

2175. **(11)** Mental Health Information 2008. The Royal College of Psychiatrists. www.rcpsych.ac.uk
page 124 All quotes from *Why Love Matters* by Sue Gerhardt (Brunner-Routledge, 2004) **(12)** p64 **(13)** p66
page 125 (14) p78 **(15)** p80 **(16)** p102 **(17)** p42 **(18)** p45 **(19)** p37 **(20)** p38 **(21)** p42
page 126 (22) p77 **(23)** p73

Ouch! Common breastfeeding complaints

page 133 (1) These chemicals are postulated as glucosinate compounds including potassium myronate (The last word, readers' letters, *New Scientist*, 19 May 2007) and the amino-acid methionone (Cabbage leaves for treatment and prevention of breast engorgement, S Smith, www.breastfeedingonline.com/cabbage)
page 136 (2) Nipple Vasospasm – a manifestation of Raynaud's phenomenon and a preventable cause of breastfeeding failure. L Lawlor-Smith, C Lawlor-Smith sourced through www.kellymom.com
page 137 (3) Dr Sears and Dr Newman both recognise the efficacy of gentian violet and recommend it as a thrush treatment despite the carcinogenic association
page 138 (4) 'The level of fluconazole passing into Breastmilk is reported as 400 microgrammes per kg per day, while the paediatric dose is 6mg per kg per day to start followed by 3mg per kg per day' (Hale, 2006). **(5)** The World Health Organisation recognises fluconazole as compatible with breastfeeding. World Health Organisation. www.breastfeedingnetwork.org.uk/pdfs/BFN_Thrush.pdf. **(6)** 'Fluconazole has also been studied in babies of <1000g born prematurely and at risk of severe fungal infections, without adverse effects, (Kaufman D et al, 2001). The safety profile of the drug may therefore be assumed to be greater than the recommendation that it should not be used during lactation suggests.' NHS Education for Scotland. www.nes.scot.nhs.uk/pharmacy/breastfeeding/topic4/fluconazole

Out and about without your baby

page 163 (1) and **(6)** The quality of different types of child care at 10 and 18 months: a comparison between types and factors related to quality. P Leach, J Barnes, LE Malmberg et al. *Early Child Development and Care*, February 2008: 178: 2: 177–209. **(2) (4) (5)** Shared care: establishing a balance between home and child care settings. L Ahnert, ME Lamb. *Child Development*, 2003: 74: 4: 1044–1049. **(3)** Penelope Leach, co-director of large-scale longditudinal study Families, Children and Child Care, quoted in 'Nursery Tales', *The Guardian*, 8 July 2004

When it's time to wean

page 186 (1) Global Strategy on Infant and Child Feeding **(2)** Why I still breastfeed my four-year-old' Annalisa Barbieri, *The Independent*, 13 November 2007. **(3)** The effects of breastfeeding on toddler health. EE Gulick. *Pediatric Nursing*, January-February 1986: 12: 1: 51-4. **(4)** Breastfeeding and cognitive function bibliography by Marsha Walker RN quoted on www.kellymom.com **(5)** Breast feeding and obesity: cross sectional study. R von Kries et al. *BMJ*, 1999: 319: 147-150. **(6)** Dewey KG. Nutrition, Growth, and Complementary Feeding of the Breastfed Infant. *Pediatric Clinics of North American*, February 2001: 48: 1 quoted on www.kellymom.com **(7)** A time to wean. KA Dettwyler. *New Beginnings*, May 1995: 12: 67-87. **(8)** Wikes 1953 quoted in *Breastfeeding: Biocultural Perspectives* by Patricia Stuart-Macadam and Katherine A Dettwyler (Aldine de Gruyter, 1995) p84
page 187 (9) Breastfeeding and subsequent social adjustment in six- to eight-year-old children. DM Ferguson. *Journal of Childrens Psychology, Psychiatry and Allied Disciplines*, 1987: 28:378-86.

Ignore this book

Guilt is the curse of parenthood. This book is meant as a funny, handy guide to helping you to enjoy your baby. Feel free to disagree with it. It's not a prescription, and you know your baby better than I do.

Don't let this book replace one set of guilty hand-wringing with another:

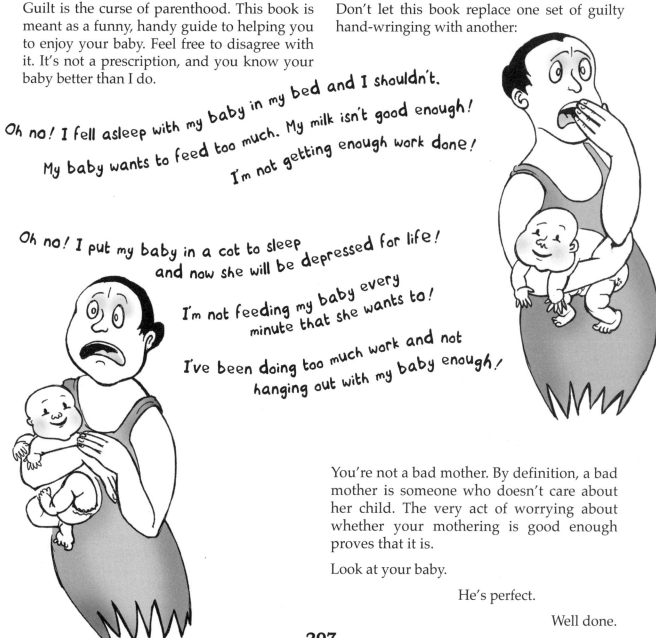

Oh no! I fell asleep with my baby in my bed and I shouldn't.

My baby wants to feed too much. My milk isn't good enough!

I'm not getting enough work done!

Oh no! I put my baby in a cot to sleep and now she will be depressed for life!

I'm not feeding my baby every minute that she wants to!

I've been doing too much work and not hanging out with my baby enough!

You're not a bad mother. By definition, a bad mother is someone who doesn't care about her child. The very act of worrying about whether your mothering is good enough proves that it is.

Look at your baby.

He's perfect.

Well done.

MORE BY KATE EVANS FROM MYRIAD

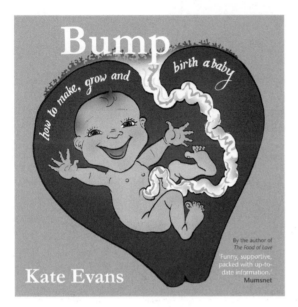

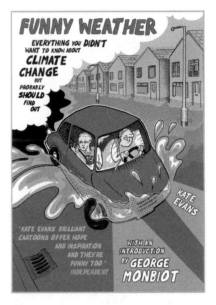

Kate Evans's ground-breaking new book on pregnancy and birth supports women in all their choices.

It includes practical help for those trying to conceive, early pregnancy advice, how to engage with the professionals, abortion rights, miscarriage support, information on screening and scans, and how to prepare for the art of birth: labour, and the Caesarean section.

'They say a picture speaks a thousand words – and that's certainly true of *Bump*, that guides you through the complex emotional roller coaster of conception, pregnancy and birth (not to mention loss) with help from witty, intelligent and sometimes graphic cartoons.'
Prima Baby Magazine

KATE EVANS'S PERENNIAL BEST-SELLER

'Kate Evans's brilliant cartoons offer hope and inspiration. And they're funny too.'
Independent

'A graphic guide to global warming that discusses some very chewy science using pictures and captions. If you think this all sounds a bit weird, you would be totally right – but then the best cartoons often are.'
Guardian

'Buy this book, read it, give it away. Then, as Kate says, better get on with it.'
New Internationalist

'Scientifically rigorous, politically and economically literate and astute, and deeply engaging at a human level.'
Ecologist

ISBN: 978-1-908434-35-7
E-ISBN: 978-1-908434-55-5
Available online at www.sequential-app.com

ISBN: 978-0-954930-93-6
Available online at www.sequential-app.com